White Cell Manual
edition 4

White Cell Manual
edition 4

DANE R. BOGGS, M.D.

Professor of Medicine
University of Pittsburgh
Pittsburgh, Pennsylvania

ALAN WINKELSTEIN, M.D.

Professor of Medicine
University of Pittsburgh
Head, Clinical Immunology Unit
Montefiore Hospital
Pittsburgh, Pennsylvania

 F. A. DAVIS COMPANY • Philadelphia

Library of Congress Cataloging in Publication Data

Boggs, Dane R.
   White cell manual.

   Bibliography: p.
   Includes index.
   1. Leucocytes.   2. Leucocyte disorders.
I. Winkelstein, Alan.   II. Title.   [DNLM: 1. Leukocytes. WH 200 B675w]
QP95.B59 1983   612′.112   82-23474
ISBN 0-8036-0961-2

PREFACE TO THE FOURTH EDITION

This manual first appeared in mimeograph form in 1967, prepared as a teaching aid for the first class of medical students at Rutgers Medical School. Some members of the informal "Hematology Teaching Club," chaired by Dr. Hale Ham, chose to use it in their introductory courses, and the first and second editions were privately printed and distributed. Dr. Alan Winkelstein assumed coauthorship responsibility for the third edition, especially for the sections dealing with immunology and the lymphocytic system.

The manual explores current concepts of the morphology of the leukocyte systems, the sites of cell production, cell distribution within the body, the life span of the cells, the function of the cells, and changes in cellular physiology which may be reflected in disease or may produce disease. Students who thoroughly understand the physiology of these cells insofar as it is presently known will be prepared to understand changes in leukocytes encountered in a variety of diseases. Portions of the manual are somewhat speculative and represent the authors' best guess as to the system.

The reader should *not* expect to find comprehensive discussions of the topics dealt with herein. The manual is designed to introduce medical students and other health science students to the normal function of the leukocytic systems and to the numerical and functional alterations in the systems associated with disease. Examples of diseases are given, but comprehensive lists of diseases affecting each component of the system are not. These can be found in the two major hematology texts or in the selected references listed at the end of the manual.

We are particularly indebted to our administrative assistants, Annette Broadus and Mary Almade. They (and we) are in turn indebted to those who developed word processing equipment with which this edition was prepared. The patience of our wives, Sallie and Ann, the advice of colleagues, and the permission of the latter to use material from their publications is greatly appreciated.

We will continue to be very appreciative of all comments and criticisms sent to us, especially from colleagues utilizing this manual in hematology-related course work.

Dane R. Boggs, M.D.
Alan Winkelstein, M.D.

CONTENTS

1

INTRODUCTION

In the blood of normal man, the following types of leukocytes may be distinguished in order of frequency: neutrophils, lymphocytes, monocytes, eosinophils, and basophils (Table 1). Lymphocytes are produced in many sites, but production of neutrophils, monocytes, eosinophils, and basophils is limited to the bone marrow in normal man. Also in bone marrow and in other sites, other types of leukocytes, such as plasma cells and macrophages, are observed.

The primary function of the entire system of leukocytes is defense against "foreignness." However, each of these types of cell, that is, neutrophils, lymphocytes, monocytes, eosinophils, and basophils, has different functions, and each behaves as a related but separate system. Therefore, it is strongly advised that the student form the habit of thinking about lymphocytes, neutrophils, and the other cells as individual types of cells, rather than about "leukocytes" as a general term.

The leukocyte systems differ from the erythroid and platelet systems in many respects. The latter two function in the blood, while the function of leukocytes is carried out extravascularly. Therefore, the blood merely serves as a street which a white cell uses to get from one place to another.

Defense against "foreignness" involves two general mechanisms: phagocytosis of substances recognized as foreign, and the development of an immune response against a foreign substance (an antigen). Lymphocytes and plasma cells are concerned with immunity, and this cellular system will be termed the "immunocyte" system. Neutrophils, monocytes, eosinophils, and basophils are

TABLE 1. Concentration of Leukocytes in Venous Blood Samples*

	Cells/mm^3	
	Mean	Normal Range
Neutrophils: White subjects	3,700	2,000–7,000
Black subjects	3,400	1,300–7,000
Lymphocytes	2,500	1,500–4,000
Monocytes	400	200–1,000
Eosinophils	150	0*–700
Basophils	30	0*–150

*Total leukocyte count (Coulter Counter) times the percentage of each cell type as determined in a 200 cell differential count of Wright's stained blood smear equals concentration of each cell type (291 normal subjects). A true zero value for eosinophils and basophils is not normal. A few always can be found if the blood truly is normal. However, the technique used for counting may yield a zero value, and this will occur more frequently when only 100 cells are enumerated in the differential examination. Many laboratories are converting to automated differential counting systems, and results obtained with these may differ somewhat from those obtained by manual methods. (From Orfanakis et al, Am J Clin Pathol 53:647, 1970, with permission.)

cells capable of phagocytosis (the phagocytic system). However, the phagocytic and immunocytic systems are highly interrelated in their functions. For example, monocytes process an antigen in a manner that initiates a lymphocytic response resulting in antibody production. In turn, neutrophils are more efficient phagocytes for bacteria that have been coated with antibody (opsonized) than for bacteria without antibody.

2

MORPHOLOGY
(LIGHT MICROSCOPY)

Although there are many morphologic features by which cells may be recognized, when all else fails the pattern of nuclear chromatin often is the most useful identifying feature. It cannot be emphasized too strongly that properly stained, thin smears of blood or bone marrow are necessary for accurate morphologic identification.

Mature neutrophils (polymorphonuclear, PMN, "segs") have a segmented nucleus with the segments separated by a filamentous strand. In Wright's stained smears, the nucleus is dark blue and the chromatin is very heavily clumped. The abundant cytoplasm is slightly pink, and dark lysosomes (granules) are "neutral" stained (specific, secondary) or pink (azurophilic, primary). Three segments is the average number, but a rare cell with as many as five segments is found in normal blood.

Band neutrophils, a slightly immature form compared with PMN, are also found in normal blood. Except for their lack of filamentous segmentation, they are otherwise similar to the PMN. Bands function about as well as PMN (migration into exudates, phagocytic efficiency). (See Fig. 15 for diagram of bands and segs.)

Metamyelocytes and other still more immature forms rarely are seen in normal blood. The nucleus is oval or bean-shaped, but with no beginning segmentation. Nuclear chromatin is distinctly clumped, but not to a degree comparable with that of the PMN; cytoplasm has a more bluish color due to the greater RNA content, but a full complement of granules is present. On blood smears, metamyelocytes and monocytes often are confused with one another.

Neutrophil precursors capable of mitotsis, which are categorized into morphologically identifiable subsets, are, in order of increasing maturity, *myeloblasts, promyelocytes,* and *myelocytes.* In all, the nucleus is round or oval. The nuclear chromatin is very fine in the myeloblasts, slightly clumped in promyelocytes, and more distinctly clumped in the myelocyte. Nucleoli are prominent in myeloblasts and promyelocytes, but less distinct in myelocytes. The cytoplasm is blue in myeloblasts and takes on an increasingly "neutral" color as the cell matures. Granules are absent in myeloblasts, but azurophilic (primary) granules are present in promyelocytes, and "specific" (secondary) granules appear at the myelocyte stage. These cells tend to be larger than metamyelocytes, but their size varies greatly. This is to be expected, since they are in a generative cycle. A cell preparing to enter mitosis should be twice as large as a cell that has just completed mitosis.

To a certain degree, the above represent somewhat arbitrary divisions of a cellular continuum and all stages of parallel maturation are not so orderly. For example, a cell may have chromatin with no clumping, suggesting a myeloblast, but a few azurophilic granules may be present, suggesting a promyelocyte. However, the actual granule development is quite orderly. All primary granules are synthesized at the promyelocyte stage, and all secondary granules at the myelocyte stage.

Eosinophils and *basophils* have the same general morphologic characteristics and developmental sequence as neutrophils. Their characteristic large, bright red (eosinophil) or deep purple (basophil) granules appear at the myelocyte stage. While precursors of eosinophils and neutrophils younger than the myelocyte cannot be distinguished from one another by light microscopy before their distinctive granules are synthesized, they can be separated at the promyelocyte stage by electron microscopy. The granules of basophils often overlie and obscure the nucleus. The number of nuclear segments in eosinophils is less than in neutrophils, more than three segments being rare; and basophils rarely contain more than two segments.

Lymphocytes vary in size from slightly larger than a red cell to as large as, or larger than, monocytes. They usually are round, with round nuclei, but both overall cell shape and nuclear shape may be oval or slightly indented, and nuclei may be deeply clefted. The cytoplasm usually is sky blue, but may be very light or very dark blue. Cytoplasm may be so scant that it is difficult to discern in small lymphocytes, but usually is abundant in larger lymphocytes. Occasionally, a few pink (azurophilic) granules are visible in the cytoplasm. Nuclear chromatin is heavily clumped, but the border between chromatin and parachromatin (clear spaces between chromatin) is less distinct than in neutrophils. Nucleoli are sometimes discernible. The actively dividing form of lymphocytes, the lymphoblast, is a large cell. In most instances of lymphoblastic leukemia, nuclear chromatin is fine, but barely detectably clumped. However, chromatin clumping usually is obvious in nonleukemic lymphoblasts ("activated lymphocytes"), which are found in the blood. Nucleoli are easily seen in either type of lymphoblast.

The plasma cell, an offspring of the lymphocyte, is not normally seen in blood smears. It bears a resemblance to the lymphocyte, and cells with features of both cells (plasmacytoid lymphocytes, lymphocytoid plasma cells) are sometimes observed. The plasma cell is round or oval with a round nucleus located eccentrically in the cell. Cell size is quite variable, and in general, the smaller the cell the deeper the blue color of the cytoplasm. There usually is a crescent-shaped, lighter-colored perinuclear clear zone. Nuclear chromatin is heavily clumped and chromatin-parachromatin borders are more distinct than in lymphocytes.

Morphologic identification of the monocyte is more difficult than for any of the foregoing cells. This is due to their great variation in morphologic appearance. The only universally reliable characteristic of the monocyte is its nuclear chromatin. The chromatin is clumped, but the clumps are smaller in diameter and more elongated than in lymphocytes or neutrophils. A lace-like (reticular) chromatin network can usually be discerned (or hallucinated). Monocytes usually are larger than neutrophils. The cell usually is round, and in some, the cytoplasmic border is wavy or has evident pseudopods. The "classic" monocyte has blue-gray cytoplasm, but it may be blue or neutral. The "classic" monocyte has very tiny, difficult-to-see granules, but they can be heavily and obviously granulated. Cytoplasmic vacuoles often are evident. The "classic" monocyte has a kidney-shaped nucleus, but the nucleus may be round or oval without indentation and may even be segmented on rare occasions. Because of this highly variable morphologic appearance, monocytes may resemble and be confused with large lymphocytes and metamyelocytes.

The macrophage, the larger and more differentiated offspring of the monocyte, rarely is found in normal blood, but is widely distributed in tissues (see page 50). Its nucleus usually is round or oval and more than one nucleus may be found in a cell, as a result of cell fusion. Nuclear chromatin is similar to that of the monocyte, but the clumping often is more distinct, emphasizing its reticular appearance. Cytoplasm is abundant and often contains vacuoles which may appear empty or may contain various types of phagocytosed debris.

3
STEM CELLS

In each of the cellular systems of blood, a significant number of cells die each day. Yet the normal number of cells within the body of an adult is relatively constant. Therefore, it is apparent that cells must be steadily replaced. The source of cell replacement is the stem cell system.

The hematopoietic stem cell system transcends the white cell system, encompassing erythrocytes and platelets, as well as certain cells not necessarily included in ordinary definitions of the hematopoietic system, such as tissue mast cells, osteoclasts, and the entire system of macrophages (histiocytes, Kupfer cells, and so forth) found in various tissues and body cavities (the reticuloendothelial system).

The mechanism for new cell production in any mammalian cellular system is the process of mitosis. That is, the amount of DNA and certain (but not all) other cell constituents is doubled and mitosis then produces two daughter cells which often are identical to the original mother cell. Capability of *self-replication* is the defining characteristic of any stem cell. The second necessary characteristic of a functional hematopoietic stem cell is *differentiation*.

Daughters of stem cells undergoing mitosis must be capable of maturation as well as being capable of retaining all the characteristics of the mother and of dividing again. Such a stem cell compartment is self-sustaining. In a steady state, for each cell that matured and therefore left the stem cell compartment, another stem cell would divide, keeping the compartment of normal size (Fig. 1).

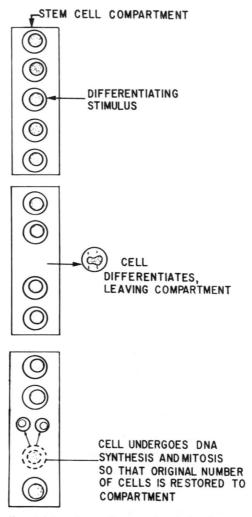

FIGURE 1. A self-sustaining stem cell compartment. An alternate model would have the differentiation stimulus trigger "asymmetric" cell division in the compartment so that mitosis of a stem would produce one stem and one differentiating cell.

Since, in all probability, each cell carries the same, or at least very similar, genetic information, one can argue that any cell within the body is theoretically a stem cell for any cellular system. The process of cellular differentiation is, in a very simplified view, a process of repression of genetic expression by the cell's genetic complement. It seems likely that when such repression and differentiation are carried beyond a certain point, cellular division for that cell is impossible. For example, there is no evidence to suggest that a mature PMN is capable of mitosis. However, there are numerous examples of cellular systems, such as hepatic cells, that ordinarily are not in mitosis, but that can be stimulated to enter mitosis. Hepatocytes are mature, well-differentiated cells with very complex and distinct metabolic functions. In the normal liver, virtually no hepatocytes are undergoing mitosis. However, if half of the liver is removed from a rodent, most remaining liver cells very quickly begin synthesizing DNA, enter mitosis, and replace the removed liver cells. Thus, the hepatocyte is a potential liver stem cell.

STRUCTURE OF THE HEMATOPOIETIC STEM CELL (HSC) SYSTEM

Basically, this consists of a complex series of concatenated compartments, each of which represents a progressive degree of differentiation, and which relate to one another as parent and progeny. Complex as it appears, the scheme portrayed in Figure 2 probably is an oversimplification of the actual system; there may be many more intermediate cells of various degrees of proliferative potential and of pluripotentiality than are shown. A still greater degree of simplification is shown in Figure 3; which we will use as a basis for illustrating certain characteristics of diseases of the HSC. None of the various HSC can be recognized as such by morphologic examination; their presence is detected by tests for cells with specialized proliferative activity (see legend for Figure 2). However, when HSC have been isolated as semi-pure cellular populations, they are medium-sized, round cells with round nuclei, fine chromatin, nucleoli, and medium blue cytoplasm; that is, really no distinguishing features. Yoffee "guessed" that a cell with such an appearance was an HSC and termed it the "transitional cell." They should *not* be referred to as "lymphocytes," as is sometimes done. A few textbooks still contain pictures of what were thought (incorrectly) to be HSC, such as "Ferrata's hemocytoblast," probably a bone marrow macrophage.

In adult life, the most primitive HSC is totipotent for *all* blood cells (see Figs. 2 and 3). The progeny of this THSC, in turn, are pluripotent for the lymphoid system and the myeloid system. Myeloid, in hematopoietic context, is properly defined as "pertaining to the bone marrow," but it will be used herein as a general term encompassing the erythroid, megakaryocyte-platelet, monocyte-macrophage, neutrophil, eosinophil, and basophil systems.

The lymphoid HSC system probably has a single cell that is capable of giving rise to the B, T, and non-B, non-T components of the system (see page 64). This pluripotent lymphoid SC (PLSC) is an immediate descendant of the THSC. In turn, there is firm proof for a separate HSC for the T cell system, a presumed direct descendant of the PLSC, and, by analogy, there is assumed to be a similar HSC for the B lymphoid compartment. In fact, each "mature" lymphocyte probably can serve as a stem cell, since under proper antigenic stimulus, it undergoes cell division, probably self-replicating. Ontogeny of the lymphoid system is discussed beginning on page 63.

Following a series of incompletely defined intermediate steps (see Fig. 2), the myeloid HSC system terminates with a series of HSC that are committed to

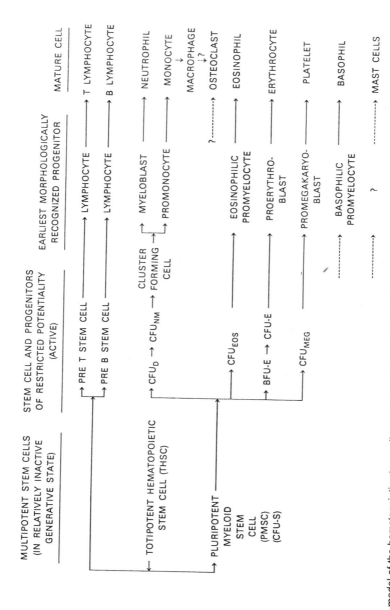

FIGURE 2. A model of the hematopoietic stem cell compartment. The undefined abbreviations refer to stem cell assays in which colonies of cells are the endpoint: CFU, colony-forming unit; S, spleen; D, diffusion chamber; NM, neutrophil-monocyte-macrophage; EOS, eosinophil; E, erythrocyte; MEG, megakaryocyte; BFU, burst-forming unit (erythroid). (From Wintrobe MM, Jee GR, Boggs DR, Bithel TC, Foerster J, Athens JW, and Jukens JN: *Clinical Hematology,* ed. 8. Lea & Febiger, Philadelphia, 1981, with permission.)

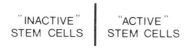

"INACTIVE" STEM CELLS | "ACTIVE" STEM CELLS

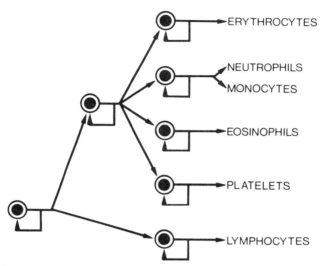

FIGURE 3. A markedly oversimplified scheme of the hematopoietic stem cell (HSC) compartment. A totipotent HSC gives rise to pluripotent myeloid and lymphoid HSC (PMHSC and PLHSC), which in turn give rise to terminal stem cell compartments.

the exclusive production of each specific type of myeloid cell (possible exception, monocytes and neutrophils may share such a "terminal" stem cell). Each such HSC can be detected by formation of colonies grown *in vitro* in semi-solid media (Table 2). These often are referred to by the nonspecific term, "progenitor" cell, and since all can be grown from bone marrow, fetal liver, and often from blood and spleen of normal man, these assays are assuming increasing importance in the study of human disease. In all probability, their overall, self-replicative, proliferative potential is much less than that of their ancestors. However, numerically, most mature cells are derived from mitoses in these terminal HSC compartments followed by non-stem-cell-type doubling divisions in the morphologically recognized mitotic compartments (Fig. 4).

An HSC compartment will normally be of stable size, reflecting the balance between self-replication and differentiation and cell death. If there is a parent compartment, as there appears to be for all but the most primitive THSC, the feed-in from the parent compartment becomes an additional variable (? primarily a back-up system for emergency use). Death and differentiation are kinetic synonyms in stem cell compartments; either event precludes self-replication. The effects of different self-replication to differentiation ratios upon HSC

TABLE 2. Methods of Assay for Definition of Hematopoietic Stem Cells

TYPE OF STEM CELL	ASSAY SYSTEM
Totipotent	Murine chimerism; lethally irradiated or congenitally anemic recipients of cells
Pluripotent myeloid	Murine chimerism; spleen colonies in irradiated recipients, in vitro "mixed" colonies*
Cell producing granulocytes and monocytes in diffusion chambers*	Cells† in cell tight diffusion chamber are implanted in an irradiated rodent
Stem cells* limited in their potentiality to: B or T lymphocytes; neutrophils and monocyte-macrophages; eosinophils; basophils; erythrocytes; megakaryocytes	Cells† added to semi-solid media in presence of appropriate stimulus, and each stem cell proliferates and its differentiated progeny form colonies. The number of colonies formed is a measure of the number of stem cells added

*Indicates that human stem cells can be analyzed; mouse is the index mammal in which all techniques were devised.
†Nucleated cells from marrow (all techniques) or from blood (most techniques).

compartment size are illustrated in Figure 5. There is some feed-in to all HSC compartments except the THSC, although it may only be intermittent. However, because of such feed-in, in the steady state, differentiation (and death) must exceed self-replication in post-THSC compartments (see Fig. 4).

Except for monocytes, macrophages, and tissue mast cells, all mature myeloid cells are end-stage cells, incapable of division. The monocyte and its progeny, the macrophage, are capable of cell division, and perhaps of self-replication (see also page 50). This is also true of other products of the HSC system, such as the mast cell. It now seems clear that "tissue" mast cells originally are derived from the HSC system. However, except under exceptional circumstances, replacement of dead tissue mast cells or an increase in their number is the result of in situ cell division, rather than the result of an influx of new cells from the blood.

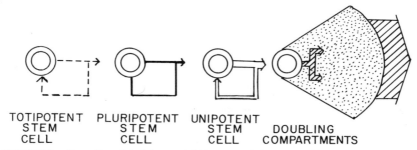

TOTIPOTENT STEM CELL   PLURIPOTENT STEM CELL   UNIPOTENT STEM CELL   DOUBLING COMPARTMENTS

FIGURE 4. Overall model of the myeloid hematopoietic system. The width of the areas indicates general rate of input and output to each compartment; dotted arrow indicates that cell ordinarily may be at rest.

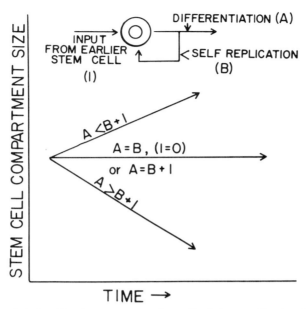

FIGURE 5. Relationship of compartment size to the balance of input, self-replication and differentiation. Refer also to Figure 4. (Courtesy of Sallie S. Boggs.)

We would emphasize that certain cells which frequently are found in abnormally large numbers in hematopoietic diseases, such as fibroblasts in the bone marrow, do *not* arise from the HSC system.

MYELOID HEMATOPOIESIS. The bone marrow is a diffusely distributed "organ" that is divisible into two general types, actively hematopoietic (red) marrow and fatty (yellow) marrow. In the newborn, most marrow is red, but by adulthood, all portions of marrow in long bones have become yellow except for patches in the heads of the humeri and femora. Red marrow has two general functions, production of new blood cells and an endocytic function. Production of new cells (hematopoiesis) occurs in the extravascular portion of the marrow. This is separated from the wide venous sinuses (intravascular marrow compartment) by a single layer of endothelial cells. This endothelial layer, which is intermittently accompanied by a discontinuous basement membrane and adjacent adventitial cells (Fig. 6), is the site of transluminal migration of mature (or maturing) blood cells and of endocytic function.

All types of blood cells are produced in the bone marrow, including lymphocytes; conversely, in normal adult man, no blood cells except lymphocytes are produced outside of the bone marrow.

EXTRAMEDULLARY HEMATOPOIESIS (EMH). As previously mentioned, myeloid hematopoiesis is limited to the bone marrow in the normal adult. In the

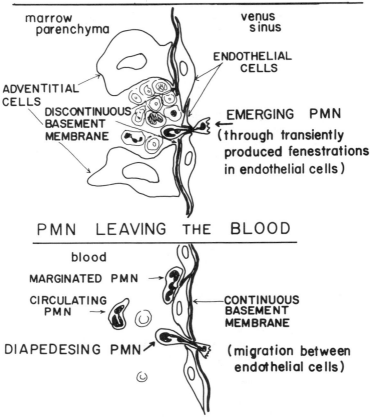

PMN ENTRANCE TO BLOOD FROM MARROW

marrow
parenchyma

venus
sinus

ENDOTHELIAL
CELLS

ADVENTITIAL
CELLS

DISCONTINUOUS
BASEMENT
MEMBRANE

EMERGING PMN
(through transiently
produced fenestrations
in endothelial cells)

PMN LEAVING THE BLOOD

blood

MARGINATED PMN →

CIRCULATING
PMN →

CONTINUOUS
BASEMENT
MEMBRANE

DIAPEDESING PMN ↗

(migration between
endothelial cells)

FIGURE 6. The structure of red bone marrow and egress of mature cells from marrow (*top*) as contrasted with egress of neutrophils from the blood (diapedesis) (*bottom*). Cells leaving the marrow parenchyma for a venous sinus do so through transient holes in endothelial cells while the neutrophil in diapedesis leaves the blood for tissue through endothelial cell junctions. (Courtesy of Sallie S. Boggs.)

embryo, hematopoiesis begins in the yolk sac, then shifts primarily to the liver, and also occurs transiently in sites such as spleen and kidney. In the full-term neonate, marrow hematopoiesis predominates. However, there is a group of rare, severe diseases, the recessively-inherited osteopetroses, in which EMH persists throughout life. The marrow cavity is virtually obliterated by excessive bone (failure of osteoclasts to resorb bone), but evidence from study of a similar disease in rodents indicates that the EMH is not due to simple "crowding out" of marrow hematopoiesis. EMH is occasionally observed in a wide spectrum of diseases, but routinely resumes during postnatal life only with diseases such as the leukemias and idiopathic myelofibrosis. Factors controlling EMH are not understood, but it does *not* occur routinely in response to prolonged and extensive demand for excess production of normal blood cells.

THE STEM CELL DISEASES

A wide variety of diseases *affect* the HSC system, influencing the quantity and/or quality of its output of differentiated hematopoietic cells. However, certain diseases are *due to* specific abnormalities of the HSC system *per se.* Principal among these are the *clonal neoplasms* of HSC. The term clonal implies that the entire tumor, or for that matter any collection of cells, is derived from a single cell.

Proof of clonality of human disease relies heavily upon the hypothesis first proposed by Lyon and now fairly well substantiated. With respect to the HSC system and clonal diseases of the HSC, "lyonization" can be summarized as follows. In the female, at a reasonably early stage of embryogenesis, one of the two X chromosomes contained in each cell is "inactivated." Inactivation is a fairly random event, so that one of the two X chromosomes is inactivated in approximately half of the cells and the other in the other half. As the embryo grows, in all descendants of each cell the same X chromosome that was originally inactivated remains so; that is, each cell "breeds true." Thus, in the adult, approximately half of the cells of any system, including the hematopoietic system, are under the influence of one of the two X chromosomes.

The gene for glucose-6-phosphate dehydrogenase (G6PD) is on the X chromosome. The common G6PD isozyme is Gd^B (B), and blacks frequently have a varient isozyme, Gd^A (A) or Gd^{A-} (A −). Approximately one third of black women are heterozygous for these enzymes, that is, have tissues in which half of the cells express A and half express B (Fig. 7). If a neoplasm begins in a single cell in such a heterozygous patient and only that cell proliferates to form a tumor (clonal) only one isozyme is expressed in the tumor (see Fig. 7). With very rare exception, all human malignant neoplasms that have been studied by this technique have been clonal. The ease with which specific, mature hematopoietic cells can be isolated and studied has led to very extensive studies of hematologic neoplasms in patients heterozygous for G6PD.

Certain types of clonal neoplasms of hematopoietic tissue are listed in Table 3, but there are many variants of these diseases and many fairly rare diseases that are more difficult to classify.

All involve an abnormal expansion of one or more hematopoietic cell compartments in the absence of any apparent stimulus for proliferation of such a cell(s). In some, the tumor cells are morphologically indistinguishable from normal cells, while in others, the cells are morphologically abnormal. The definition of certain commonly used terms, such as "leukemia," "lymphoma," "chronic," and "acute," is somewhat arbitrary but is of value in describing the natural course of the diseases and in choosing therapy and predicting response to therapy. The term *leukemia* is not restricted to its literal meaning of white blood. In the case of the chronic leukemias, leukocytosis is a requisite for diagnosis. However, a diagnosis of acute leukemia is made in the absence of leukocytosis

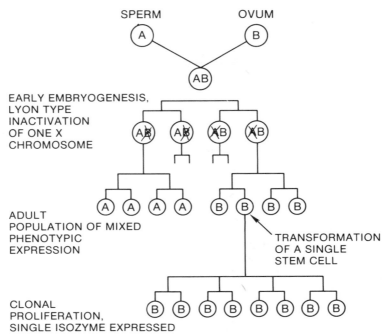

SPERM   OVUM

EARLY EMBRYOGENESIS,
LYON TYPE
INACTIVATION
OF ONE X
CHROMOSOME

ADULT
POPULATION OF MIXED
PHENOTYPIC
EXPRESSION

TRANSFORMATION
OF A SINGLE
STEM CELL

CLONAL
PROLIFERATION,
SINGLE ISOZYME EXPRESSED

FIGURE 7. Schematic representation of the basis for the use of G6PD analysis in isozymic heterozygotes in determining clonal origin of neoplasms. A indicates the isozyme Gd^A or Gd^{A-} and B indicates Gd^B. (From Wintrobe MM, Jee GR, Boggs DR, Bithel TC, Foerster J, Athens JW, and Jukens JN: *Clinical Hematology*, ed. 8. Lea & Febiger, Philadelphia, 1981, with permission.)

in approximately 40 percent of patients. When the total white blood cell count is normal or low (leukopenia) in patients with acute leukemia, immature cells usually are still present in a high percentage on differential leukocyte counts ("subleukemic leukemia"). Occasionally, leukopenia is present and no immature cells are found ("aleukemic leukemia"); examination of the bone marrow discloses an abundance of immature cells and this plus other typical clinical and laboratory features leads to the correct diagnosis. *Acute* and *chronic* were very apt descriptive terms with respect to expected survival before "modern" therapy was developed. Presently, many patients with acute lymphoblastic leukemia are cured and even those who are not cured often live longer than do patients with chronic myeloid leukemia. However, acute and chronic still are *apropos* with respect to the rapidity of onset of the diseases and for dictating the aggressiveness of therapy. *Lymphoma* is a general term applied to tumors that usually begin in lymph nodes. However, lymphomas may seemingly begin in and even be limited to non-lymph-node sites of lymphopoiesis, such as thymus, Peyer's patches, spleen, or bone marrow. At times, the clinical distinctions between various diseases listed in Table 3 are a bit fuzzy. However, even though they seemingly may "progress" from one to another or present with features of more

TABLE 3. Selected Clonal Neoplasms of Hematopoietic Tissue

PRIMARY CELLULAR EXPRESSION	APPROXIMATE MEDIAN DURATION OF *UNTREATED* SURVIVAL FROM DIAGNOSIS
Myeloid	
Leukemia	
Chronic myeloid leukemia (CML)	4 years
Acute myeloid leukemia (AML)	2 months
Lymphoma	
Hodgkin's disease* (HD)	? 3 years
Polycythemia vera (PV)	10 years
Idiopathic myelofibrosis (IMF)	5 years
Paroxysmal nocturnal hemoglobinuria (PNH)	long but unknown
Lymphoid	
Leukemia	
Chronic lymphocytic leukemia (CLL)	5 + years
Acute lymphoblastic leukemia (ALL)	3 months
Lymphoma†	
Reasonably well-differentiated lymphocytic lymphomas	5 + years
Less well-differentiated lymphocytic lymphomas	<1 year
Multiple myeloma (MM)	? 2 years

*Current evidence indicates that the "neoplastic" cell in this disease is at least a close relative of the monocyte-macrophage system and that the characteristic lymphocytic infiltration is "reactive."
†A bewildering array of subclassification of what has been termed "non-Hodgkin's lymphoma" is available.

than one disease, specific diagnoses are desirable. Thus, we discourage the use of the broad (but nondiagnostic) terms of "myeloproliferative" and "lymphoproliferative" disorders. These often are used to encompass CML, AML, PV, and IMF ("myeloproliferative"), and CLL, ALL, lymphomas, and MM ("lymphoproliferative"). Three examples of difficult or even impossible differential diagnoses are as follows. (1) CML usually terminates in "blast crisis" in which case the overall clinical picture may be identical to an acute leukemia. However, response to therapy of the blast crisis of CML is inferior to response to appropriate therapy for the respective type of acute leukemia that is being mimicked. (2) Patients with PV may develop severe degrees of myelofibrosis and, except for the history of preceding PV, are indistinguishable from IMF. (3) Patients whose principal manifestation of well-differentiated lymphocytic lymphoma is infiltration of the bone marrow cannot be distinguished from CLL except for the absence of increased lymphocytes in blood. However, terming such patients "aleukemic CLL" may be inappropriate, since their prognosis is distinctly inferior to that of patients with CLL.

The nature of the defects in the tumor forming HSC is unknown, but it clearly differs from disease to disease. In the myeloid stem cell diseases listed in Table 3, the abnormal stem cell completely overgrows the normal myeloid HSC system so that all cells produced are part of the clone. However, in most instances, normal HSC still are present but are at rest (Fig. 8). The abnormal HSC must have a growth advantage relative to the normal HSC. It does not necessarily grow more rapidly than normal. In fact, the situation that is discussed for CML, an expanded (but abnormal) proliferative compartment with a slower than normal generation time, usually prevails. The old notion that leukemia (or cancer in general) represents abnormally rapid cell growth has proved to be incorrect.

Tumor cells generally are capable of responding to certain normal growth stimuli, but at the same time are relatively autonomous; that is, they will grow without evident stimulation or with virtually undetectable levels of stimulus. For example, the principal expression of PV is erythrocytosis (see section on PV below). Normally, colonies of erythroid cells grown *in vitro* require erythropoietin for growth. Erythropoietin stimulation is the primary means by which normal red cell production is controlled *in vivo*. In PV, colonies will grow without addition of erythropoietin to the culture, but more colonies grow if the hormone is added (autonomous but responsive). In fact, the stem cell probably is not really autonomous, but rather is responding to very low levels of erythropoietin; addition of an antibody directed against erythropoietin abolishes growth.

TOTAL STEM CELL POOL SIZE

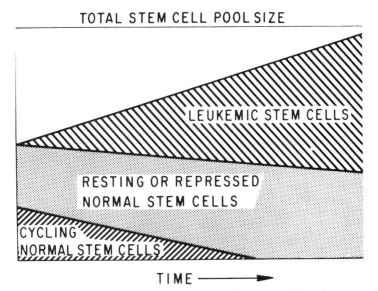

FIGURE 8. Model for clonal growth of an abnormal stem cell. Normal stem cells are initially repressed (mechanism unknown) and they may disappear eventually.

SPECIFIC DISEASES. Throughout this manual we will refer to these neoplasms as examples regarding certain hematopoietic changes, but in this brief section we will give a capsule summary of certain "index" types of diseases. All of these diseases are more common in men than in women, the male:female ratio ranging from approximately 4:3 for ALL to approximately 2:1 for CLL. CLL and MM are diseases primarily of "old age" and almost never are observed before age 30. Conversely, the peak incidence of ALL is at age 3, and by age 40 it becomes uncommon. CML, AML, HD, and lymphoid lymphomas occur at any age but become increasingly frequent as age advances. The same is true for PV and IMF, although both are rare in childhood.

Therapy is generally beyond the scope of this manual. However, we would note that *cure* is the expected result of complex and rather toxic therapy in at least two thirds of patients with HD and half of the children (but not adults) with ALL. Occasional cures are affected in AML and in certain specific types of lymphoid lymphomas. Conversely, cure is not a reasonable goal in patients with CLL, CML, MM, PV, IMF, PNH, and in most varieties of lymphoid lymphomas. When cure is a reasonable goal or if a remission will prolong useful life to a significant degree (as in AML), severely toxic therapy can be justified. Noncurative therapy associated with modest, transient, iatrogenic illness is tolerable as therapy designed to relieve symptoms in the other diseases. Many of us believe that no specific antitumor therapy can be justified in most patients with IMF and PNH or in patients with CLL and certain forms of lymphoid lymphoma in whom only modest or no symptoms are present.

Chronic Myeloid Leukemia (CML)

The principal feature of CML (chronic [myelogenous, granulocytic, myelocytic] leukemia) is increased mature neutrophils in blood (neutrophilia) accompanied by the entire spectrum of neutrophil precursors normally found only in bone marrow. However, in many patients, blood levels of platelets, monocytes, eosinophils, basophils, and even lymphocytes are increased. Conversely, red cell production is decreased, resulting in anemia. The patient's principal complaint is fatigue, reflecting not only anemia, but also "hypermetabolism" secondary to the metabolic imposition of the tumor. Abnormal physical findings usually are limited to pallor, splenomegaly, and sternal tenderness (a spot of often exquisite tenderness most often in the midbody of the sternum). The chronic phase of the disease is brought under control and kept under control by relatively simple and nontoxic therapy with busulfan. However, "blast crisis" can and does develop at any time (may be present at onset or be delayed in rare patients for more than 20 years) and is the cause of death in at least 80 percent of patients. The clinical pattern of blast crisis usually mimics AML, but may show features of ALL.

The hallmark of CML is the Philadelphia chromosome (Ph'). This is an acquired chromosome defect and is recognized by a shortening of the long arms of chromosome #22. This is due to translocation, usually from chromosome #22 to #9, but sometimes to other chromosomes. Patients who appear to have CML but who do not have the Ph¹ defect have a much poorer prognosis than does the Ph¹⁺ patient. The Ph¹ is found routinely in precursors of all myeloid cells, but usually is not found in lymphocytes. At least certain populations of lymphocytes *are* part of the clone as determined by G6PD studies and, as noted above, a lymphoid blast crisis can occur. Therefore, if a cell has a Ph¹ defect, it is part of the clone; but if it does not, it still may be leukemic, that is, the chromosome defect marks the clone but does not necessarily encompass it. This also is true in the acute leukemias and the concept is illustrated in Figure 9.

From the above, it seems evident that CML begins as a clonal disease of a totipotent HSC, feeding cells into any or all blood cell compartments (Fig. 10). Increased production is responsible for the increased number of cells, but this reflects an increase in overall number of precursor cells which, in fact, have a slower than normal generation time (Fig. 11). This expanded production compartment is producing cells in a fairly normal fashion and the cells which are produced are not particularly abnormal. The mature cells usually have one demonstrable chemical defect, a decreased leukocyte alkaline phosphatase (LAP). Reduced LAP of mature neutrophils is quite helpful in distinguishing CML from other causes of neutrophilia ("leukemoid reactions").

There is also a distinct abnormality in cellular release in this disease, in that immature cells are released to the blood. It is rare to see more than an occasional metamyelocyte in the blood of nonleukemic patients. However, in CML many immature cells are released to the blood and the same spectrum of cells is seen in the blood that is seen in the bone marrow. In all probability, this is not a primary defect of the disease because the occasional patient who is examined when the disease is in a very early stage usually has only mature neutrophils in the blood.

Acute Myeloid Leukemia (AML)

This probably is the most "malignant" of all human neoplasms, in that untreated patients may die within a few days of diagnosis and their median survival is

◯ Clone

◌ Chromosomally abnormal cells

◉ Morphologically identifiable cells

FIGURE 9. Interrelationship of a clone of tumor cells to morphologically identifiable cells of the clone and of cells in the clone with chromosomal abnormalities. Studies in CML and in the acute leukemias form the basis for the various relationships that are portrayed. (From Wintrobe MM, Jee GR, Boggs DR, Bithel TC, Foerster J, Athens JW, and Jukens JN: *Clinical Hematology*, ed. 8. Lea & Febiger, Philadelphia, 1981, with permission.)

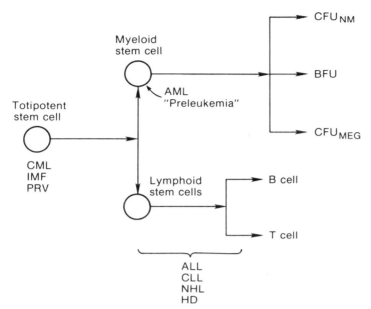

FIGURE 10. The possible site of stem cell origin of various leukemias and related diseases. The structure of the hematopoietic stem cell compartment is shown as an overly simplified model. Abbreviations: CFU_{NM}, colony-forming unit producing neutrophils and macrophages; BFU, burst-forming unit producing erythrocytes; CFU_{MEG}, colony-forming unit producing megakaryocytes. (From Wintrobe MM, Jee GR, Boggs DR, Bithel TC, Foerster J, Athens JW, and Jukens JN: *Clinical Hematology*, ed. 8. Lea & Febiger, Philadelphia, 1981, with permission.)

only two months. Rapid, sudden death usually is observed in those whose leukocyte count is rising very rapidly. In this circumstance, the leukemic cells lodge and grow in small vessels, particularly those of the brain, forming macroscopic tumors which in turn lead to sudden, massive, intracerebral hemorrhage. The principal causes of morbidity and mortality in other patients are neutropenia (bacterial and fungal infection), thrombocytopenia (purpura, fatal subarachnoid and/or gastrointestinal bleeding), and anemia (fatigue). Physical findings are pallor, petechiae and ecchymoses, fever (which may be due to the disease or may reflect a complicating infection), and sternal tenderness. In approximately half of the patients, the spleen and/or the liver are enlarged. AML probably is a disease of the pluripotent, myeloid HSC (see Fig. 10). A shift to a lymphoblastic picture rarely occurs, as one might expect if it originated in the totipotent HSC, but *all* myeloid descendants of the HSC usually are involved. One major defect in this leukemic HSC is its failure to differentiate. The morphologic expression of the immature cells is highly variable. Most often, cells resembling normal myeloblasts predominate, but any myeloid precursor may be the predominant cell or may be present in increased numbers along with myeloblasts. These are immature erythroblasts (erythroleukemia, DiGuglielmo's syndrome), immature

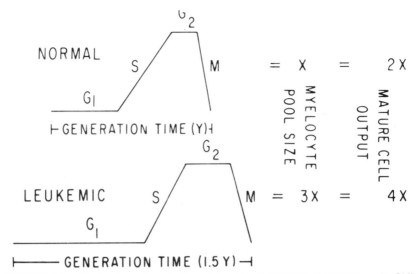

FIGURE 11. Mechanism of production of increased numbers of neutrophils in CML. Generation time (Y) is longer than normal, which slows production rate, but the number of myelocytes is increased (X), so that an overall increase in production occurs.

monocytes (acute monocytic leukemia), cells with features of myeloblasts and monocytes (acute myelomonocytic leukemia), promyelocytes (acute promyelocytic leukemia), or the cells may be very young megakaryocyte precursors (acute megakaryoblastic leukemia). When the cells are promyelocytes they may have very large, abnormal-appearing granules and these may be eosinophilic (acute eosinophilic leukemia) or even basophilic (acute basophilic leukemia). Thus, on the basis of the predominating morphologic picture, AML can be divided into at least seven diseases. However, there are no clinical differences of major importance among these, so AML can be thought of as a single disease but with variable morphologic expression. *Auer rods* are pathognomonic of AML or for CML terminating in an AML-like picture. Auer rods are abnormal primary granules and therefore pink-staining with Romanofsky stains, and are filamentous, spindle-shaped or oval rather than round.

Immature cells accumulate while production of morphologically mature erythroid and granulocytic cells and platelets is decreased, usually to a marked degree. Virtually all myeloid production is from the leukemic clone. Normal HSC are still present and regrow if remission is induced but apparently are at rest (see Fig. 8) with active disease.

Current therapy induces severe toxicity. The patient must be rendered "aplastic" by complex combinations of chemotherapeutic drugs. If supportive therapy then allows survival through this aplastic period (usually 3 to 5 weeks), normal HSC usually "re-awaken" and repopulate the system and a *complete remission* (CR) is achieved. A CR is defined in simple terms in this and in other neoplastic diseases: no evidence of tumor can be found and, with the exception of complications induced by therapy, the patient is asymptomatic. Unfortunately, in order to induce a CR in AML, patients must be made worse before they get better, and sometimes are killed. With maintenance therapy with anti-leukemic drugs, the first CR has a median duration of about a year and a few (? approximately 5 to 20 percent) are cured. The principal reason that therapy is effective in this disease (and in many others) is that normal HSC grow more rapidly than do tumor cells (see section on cytotoxic therapy and HSC).

Acute Lymphoblastic Leukemia (ALL)

Except for the morphology of the cells and the presence of more prominent enlargement of lymphoid tissue, this disease is very similar to AML with respect to signs and symptoms, but is quite dissimilar in terms of response to therapy and prognosis. This may be a disease of the pluripotent lymphoid HSC or perhaps of more restricted HSC. As noted later (see page 89), a few patients have lymphoblasts with surface and antigenic characteristics of mature T or B cells, but most do not. However, the presence of the Ia-like antigen suggests that most are in the B-cell lineage. Normal myeloid HSC are present, but their output of mature cells is reduced, resulting in the anemia, neutropenia, and thrombocytopenia seen in virtually all patients. However, the leukemic lymphoblasts do not necessarily repress normal lymphocyte function, for until patients with ALL are treated, their immune system is fairly normal.

In ALL, there are three drugs which are relatively specific for the leukemic lymphoblasts, generally sparing normal cells, including normal HSC. Thus, induction of CR with prednisone or other adrenal glucocorticosteroids and vincristine with or without added L-asparaginase does not necessarily make the patient worse during therapy. These drugs, used in combination, induce a CR in more than 90 percent of children with ALL and in a slightly smaller percentage of adults. However, they are of no benefit in maintaining remission. For that purpose, generally cytotoxic agents, usually methotrexate and 6-mercaptopurine, are utilized. A high percentage of patients with ALL have microscopic foci of lymphoblasts in the meninges. These are protected from exposure to all of the above drugs, except prednisone, by the blood-brain pharmacokinetic barrier. Unless these foci are eradicated by "prophylactic" therapy with intrathecal methotrexate or cranio-spinal radiation therapy, relapse with "meningeal" leukemia will terminate CR in months (or even years) in at least half of the patients.

However, if children with ALL are carefully and expertly treated, induced into CR, given prophylactic therapy against meningeal disease, and given maintenance chemotherapy for 2 to 3 years, at least half are cured. Unfortunately, only an occasional adult with ALL is cured with this regimen.

Polycythemia Vera (PV)

This is a fairly "benign" neoplasm probably involving the totipotent HSC (see Fig. 10). The principal expression is erythrocytosis, but all other myeloid cells tend to be increased as well. Indeed, one of the most helpful means of differentiating PV from secondary forms of polycythemia is the neutrophilia, thrombocytosis, and/or basophilia which frequently accompany PV. Erythropoietin levels are normal or decreased in PV while secondary polycythemia is due to excessive erythropoietin stimulation. The relative autonomy of PV erythroid precursors with respect to erythropoietin has been discussed (page 18). Except for splenomegaly and "plethora," the physical examination usually is unremarkable. The morphologic appearance of mature blood cells and their precursors is entirely normal in uncomplicated disease. Erythrocytosis is controlled by bleeding, or if thrombocytosis is prominent (posing a modest hazard for either hemorrhage or thrombosis), both are controlled by administration of DNA-seeking radioactive phosphorus or by other chemotherapeutic agents. Properly-treated patients usually remain asymptomatic for many years, eventually dying of complications of secondary myelofibrosis, development of an acute leukemia-like picture, seemingly unrelated causes, and so forth. The fact that the occasional patient who dies with a picture similar to acute leukemia can mimic either AML or ALL is the principal reason for suggesting that this is a disease of the totipotent HSC rather than the pluripotent myeloid HSC.

Hodgkin's Disease (HD)

This "lymphoma" is defined by the presence of Reed-Sternberg cells (RSC). The RSC resembles a macrophage and indeed has many macrophage-like functional, antigenic, and surface characteristics. Although other presumably malignant "histiocytes" are also present, the RSC is defined as a binucleated cell with a single, very large nucleolus in each nucleus. The natural course of the disease is highly variable and is very dependent upon the clinical extent of the disease (how many node groups are involved and are organs other than lymph nodes involved?) and upon histologic subclassification. As is discussed later (see page 95), T-cell function is remarkably abnormal in HD, in part, secondary to macrophage dysfunction.

Cure is the objective of therapy in all newly-diagnosed patients and in those who relapse after the first, and often after the second, curative attempt. Unlike the case of many carcinomas, surgical excision has no therapeutic role in curing limited disease. Radiotherapy is used in initial attempts to cure patients with limited disease. For patients with more extensive disease, complex combinations of chemotherapeutic agents are used, or chemotherapeutic agents and radiotherapy (combined modality therapy).

Paroxysmal Nocturnal Hemoglobinuria

This is a rare, acquired, myeloid HSC disease, but it is of particular interest in that it is the only such disease in which a chimeric population of normal and abnormal mature blood cells may coexist routinely. There is a defective membrane in cells of the abnormal clone, present in neutrophils and platelets, as well as red cells. The affected population of red cells is exceedingly sensitive to complement-associated, intravascular lysis, but in most patients, a nonsensitive and presumably normal population of red cells also is present. The disease is characterized by severe hemolysis of the affected red cells. Since complement-mediated hemolysis primarily takes place within the circulation, large amounts of free hemoglobin are filtered by the kidney with resultant hemoglobinuria.

Aplastic Anemia (AA)

This is a term used to describe a group of diseases characterized by pancyto-penia (defined as anemia, neutropenia, and thrombocytopenia) in the presence of an "empty," or at least hypoplastic, bone marrow and in the absence of any underlying causative illness. AA can be congenital (Fanconi's anemia) or acquired. The acquired forms can be secondary to idiosyncratic reactions to drugs (chloramphenicol, phenylbutazone) or toxins (benzene), viruses (hepatitis), or can be idiopathic. A form of AA is routinely induced by drugs or agents which have dose-dependent cytotoxicity (cancer therapy), but recovery from this usually is rapid and the term AA usually is not applied to this situation of transient aplasia. In chronic forms of AA, defective production of cells by the myeloid HSC compartment is present, but the exact nature of the defect is variable and poorly defined. In some, the stem cell itself appears to be abnormal. This is the group of patients that can be cured by simple infusion of marrow from an unaffected, identical twin (see discussion below). In others, there is evidence that the myeloid HSC system is being suppressed by a population of lymphocytes.

If aplasia is severe and associated with severe neutropenia (less than 500 per mm^3) and thrombocytopenia (less than 20,000 per mm^3), death usually occurs within a few weeks or months from infection and/or hemorrhage. If aplasia is less severe, patients may live for many years with waxing, waning, or even quite stable disease. However, unless recovery occurs shortly after diagnosis, complete recovery is unusual (unless a marrow transplant proves successful; see discussion below).

MARROW TRANSPLANTATION

The most widely used therapeutic application of results of research relative to HSC is transplantation of bone marrow. At present, this is the treatment of choice for certain, carefully-selected groups of patients with leukemia and aplastic anemia, as well as for patients with a variety of rare, otherwise fatal, congenital diseases due to abnormal HSC.

The crash program that led to the development of the atomic bomb was succeeded by a crash program to try to understand and subvert the morbidity and mortality induced with large doses of x- or gamma-irradiation. Three general modes of death from increasing doses of whole-body irradiation were recognized: (1) hematopoietic, in which death from infection (neutropenia) and/or bleeding (thrombocytopenia) follows interruption of cell production in the marrow; (2) gastrointestinal, in which death with fulminant, bloody diarrhea due to denudation of small intestine mucosa follows a slightly larger dose and occurs earlier than hematopoietic death; and (3) central nervous system death, which reflects complete failure of function within hours (or less) of receiving a massive dose. Jacobson observed that mice could be protected from hematopoietic death if given spleen cells shortly after irradiation. Subsequent studies indicated that HSC in marrow (or in the spleen) of mice would "home" to the marrow when given intravenously to irradiated mammals, and would reconstitute the hematopoietic system in time to prevent death. This was a highly effective form of therapy if done with inbred strains of mice (syngeneic), but much less effective with outbred strains (allogeneic).

Shortly thereafter (late 1950s), trials of marrow transplantation in humans with leukemia and aplastic anemia were undertaken, with predictable results. It was effective in a few syngeneic (identical twin) transplants, but ineffective in the allogeneic situation. In the ensuing decade, some understanding of histocompatibility loci evolved, first in the mouse (the H2 genetic loci), then in the dog (the DLA [dog leukocyte antigen] system), and then in man (the HLA [human leukocyte antigen] system), and formed a rational basis for choosing allogeneic transplant donor-recipient pairs.

It must be emphasized that marrow transplantation is conceptually different from transplantation of certain other organs, such as the kidney. The only thing asked of the transplanted kidney is that enough of it survives in the recipient to provide adequate renal function. With marrow, a tiny fraction of the organ is asked to regrow to a normal size and then keep on growing for the rest of the patient's life. Furthermore, the allogeneic marrow transplant carries lymphocytes that recognize the host as foreign and can induce fatal graft-versus-host disease (GVHD).

Three types of marrow transplantation now are utilized as therapy: autologous, syngeneic, and allogeneic. *Autologous* simply means that marrow is taken from the individual, stored (HSC retain viability when frozen under exacting conditions) and re-infused after the patient has received a very large dose of cytotoxic therapy (for various cancers). If one of a pair of *identical twins (syngeneic)* has acquired aplastic anemia, simple infusion of marrow from the normal twin usually is curative. Failure to cure in this circumstance is thought to mean that the host is attacking his own stem cells (immune suppression) (see page 69). If one twin has leukemia, or another type of cancer which is very responsive to chemotherapy, syngeneic marrow transplantation is the treatment of choice. Massive doses of cytotoxic therapy are given to eradicate the leukemic clone and marrow is infused, often inducing cures.

Allogeneic Transplantation

This is more complex than autologous or syngeneic transplantation, since measures must be taken to avoid rejection and GVH. Thomas (University of Washington, Seattle) and his coworkers have been the pioneers of marrow transplantation. Conceptually, it is a fairly simple and straightforward procedure as outlined below. In execution, each step must be managed with meticulous detail.

The proper patient must be chosen. Since the procedure itself kills a significant number of patients, the patient must be expected to die of the disease in a relatively brief time. Further, marrow transplantation should offer a reasonably good possibility of cure. For example, these criteria are met by relatively young patients with severe aplastic anemia and with certain forms and stages of leukemia; any patient with AML; patients with ALL in whom proper, initial therapy proved not to be curative; and those in the blast crisis phase of CML.

A reasonably histocompatible donor must be available (HLA matched, see page 96). Ordinarily, this will be a sibling; there is a one in four chance of any two siblings being compatible.

The recipient's immune system must be destroyed or the transplant will be rejected. This is done with potentially lethal doses of cancer chemotherapy drugs (usually cyclophosphamide) and/or whole body gamma- or x-irradiation. With leukemia, the tumor must also be destroyed, and potentially supra-lethal doses of cytotoxins are given.

Marrow is aspirated repeatedly from the anesthetized donor until at least 10^8 nucleated cells per kg of recipient's weight are obtained. The aspirated marrow is passed through a coarse filter to remove large clumps of cells and bone chips, and is given intravenously.

The recipient will then become even more neutropenic and thrombocytopenic than before the cytotoxins were given. Intensive supportive therapy is required for 2 to 4 weeks until the transplant begins to supply mature cells to the blood.

GVHD is a hazard for those who do not reject the transplant and who also survive the immediate post-transplant period. Various drugs are given to attempt to prevent and, if necessary, to treat GVHD, but as many as one fourth of transplant recipients still die from this complication.

Reconstitution of the immune system by the transplanted cells can require a year or more, so patients are at risk for potentially fatal "opportunistic" infections, such as cytomegalovirus disease.

However, if a recipient is alive and well a year after transplant, permanent cure of the disease being treated usually has been achieved.

STEM CELLS AND ANTITUMOR DRUGS

The use of cell-poisoning chemotherapeutic drugs is an important form of therapy in many forms of cancer. Ideally, one tries to poison the tumor without poisoning the host's normal cells. Unfortunately, most presently useful forms of cancer chemotherapy kill normal cells as well as cancer cells. Thus, a tightrope is walked between antitumor effect and life-threatening toxicity.

The concept of "resting," immature, stem cell compartments and actively proliferating, more mature, stem cell compartments (see Fig. 3) becomes important in understanding the nature and duration of toxicity of various classes of antitumor agents.

Cycle active agents (mitotic inhibitors, such as vinblastine and vincristine; agents killing cells only if they are in DNA synthesis, such as folic acid antagonists, cytosine arabinoside, and hydroxyurea) are drugs which kill cells that are in a generative cycle but spare resting cells. If a single dose of one of these drugs is given, then the more mature, often terminal compartments are affected, but more pluripotent compartments are spared (see Fig. 3). Thus, mature compartments can be quickly replenished from undamaged immature compartments. A patient with Hodgkin's disease given a single dose of vinblastine may develop a transient decrease in neutrophils, but the damage is usually repaired within 10 days.

Noncycle active agents (x- and gamma-irradiation, alkylating agents such as nitrogen mustard and busulfan) damage resting cells as well as cells in a generative cycle. Thus, both mature and immature stem cell compartments are affected by these agents. Damage to both compartments must be repaired before normal cell production is resumed. For example, a patient with Hodgkin's disease given a single dose of nitrogen mustard may remain neutropenic for three to four times as long as a patient given vinblastine.

4

THE PHAGOCYTE SYSTEM (NEUTROPHILS, MONOCYTES, EOSINOPHILS, BASOPHILS)

The localization and killing of invading microorganisms is the primary useful role of the phagocytic system. The formation of an inflammatory exudate, composed primarily of neutrophils and monocytes, occurs rapidly in response to a local infection or to noninfectious challenges, such as the formation of urate crystals in a gouty joint or in response to sterile tissue necrosis. Occasional eosinophils and basophils appear promptly in inflammatory exudates, but except in certain types of "allergic" disease, their numbers are small and their specific roles unknown.

When faced with foreign material, be it a bacterium, a fungus, or a glass bead, the phagocyte will ingest and attempt to destroy the material. Certain body constituents also are recognized as foreign under certain circumstances. Dead cells, probably of any variety, are recognized as foreign and can be phagocytized, usually not by PMNs but by macrophages.

NEUTROPHILS

The neutrophil is the most common cell in the bone marrow and the most common leukocyte found in the blood. However, within the entire organism there probably are more lymphocytes and as many or more monocyte-macrophages as there are neutrophils. The only proven *useful* role for the neutrophil is in preventing invasion by pathogenic microorganisms or localizing and killing them after they have invaded. The life cycle of the neutrophil can be divided into a series of compartments: production in bone marrow; storage in bone marrow; transit through the blood; egress from blood into body cavities and tissues, and egress from blood into inflammatory exudates.

Neutrophil Kinetics

A total leukocyte count and a differential leukocyte count are routinely done on the blood of any patient who is admitted to most university hospitals. If the concentration of neutrophils in blood is found to be increased, most physicians assume that production of neutrophils is increased; if the concentration of neutrophils is decreased, most physicians assume production of neutrophils is decreased. Both of these assumptions are often incorrect.

BLOOD NEUTROPHILS

Early in the 19th century, a number of physicians and physiologists observed that leukocytes within the vascular system were not all circulating freely. This has been confirmed by labeling neutrophils with radioactive substances and determining their distribution within the blood. Approximately half of the neutrophils within the confines of the blood vessels are stuck to the walls of blood vessels or are rolling along their walls, and only half are circulating freely. From a practical viewpoint, this means that if one determines the total number of freely circulating neutrophils in a sample of blood, this does not represent a sample of total blood neutrophils, but only about half of them. Marginated neutrophils may be found on any capillary or postcapillary venule, but they are particularly common in lungs, liver, and spleen. If all the neutrophils are demarginated from vessel walls into the freely circulating blood, the neutrophil count will double. Conversely, neutropenia may occur due to an increase in the proportion of cells in the blood which are marginated. These are not static compartments, for cells are exchanging rapidly and steadily between the circulating and marginal pool.

In the model of neutrophil kinetics that we develop in this section, the blood will be diagramed as a square, and the proportionate size of the circulating pool and the marginal pool will be denoted by the position of the dotted line in the square (Fig. 12). The arrows pointing in each direction indicate that cells within the circulating and marginal compartments of the blood are freely and rapidly exchanging at all times.

Normally, the rate at which new cells are entering the blood from the bone marrow and the rate at which cells are being lost to the tissues is equal. If blood from a normal subject is removed, labeled with radioactive diisopropylfluorophosphate (DF^{32}P), and returned to the same subject, one can follow the disappearance of PMN from the blood. This disappearance is a straight line when plotted semilogarithmically (Fig. 13).

The disappearance curve is exponential, that is, cells are disappearing randomly. This is in contrast to curves of DF^{32}P-labeled red cells. Red cells normally leave the blood because they die of old age. PMN leave the blood

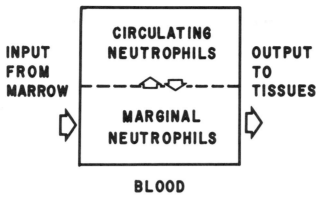

FIGURE 12. Kinetics of blood neutrophils.

presumably because there is a demand for them in tissues, body cavities, or inflamed areas, and the demand does not distinguish between relatively young or old cells. Thus, a cell that has just entered the blood from the bone marrow is as likely to leave as is a cell that has been circulating for some hours. The half disappearance time from the blood of labeled PMN averages about 7 hours. From mathematical considerations, this indicates that the average neutrophil spends 10 hours in the blood and means that the total number of neutrophils in

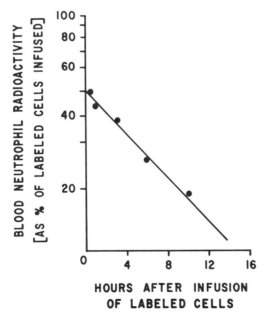

FIGURE 13. Results of studies of blood neutrophils labeled with radioactive diisopropylfluorophosphate. Blood is removed, labeled, and reinfused into the same subject.

the blood is replaced from the bone marrow approximately 2½ times each day. Again, you should contrast this with the erythrocytic mass whose cells live for an average of 120 days in the blood, and thus erythroid tissue is replaced on an average once in 120 days. In normal subjects, there is no evidence that neutrophils ever return to the bone marrow from the blood. Therefore, this system should be thought of as a one-way street. An overall model of neutrophil kinetics is shown in Figure 14.

Normally, neutrophils leave the blood to appear in bronchial washings, urine, and the gut. We do not know whether or not this accounts for most cells leaving the blood in the normal subject, and have, as yet, been unable to quantitate the importance of the sites of cell loss from the blood.

NEUTROPHIL PRODUCTION AND STORAGE

Neutrophils and neutrophil precursors in marrow can be divided into those that are capable of mitosis, and those not capable of mitosis; the mitotic (production) pool, and the postmitotic maturation and storage pool. Following feed-in from the stem cell, there is a steady continuum of maturation from the earliest recognizable precursor, the myeloblast, to the mature segmented neutrophil (PMN). However, as previously noted, this continuum has been somewhat arbitrarily divided into certain cellular subcompartments. The mitotic pool is divided into myeloblasts, promyelocytes, and myelocytes. The postmitotic maturation and storage pool is divided into metamyelocytes, bands, and segmented neutrophils. This pool is termed "postmitotic" for the obvious reason that mitosis is no longer taking place, "maturation" because a steady process of maturation is taking place within it, and "storage" because bands and segmented neutrophils can be released from this pool to the blood upon demand. Normally, the average cell spends approximately 10 days in the maturation and storage pool. The

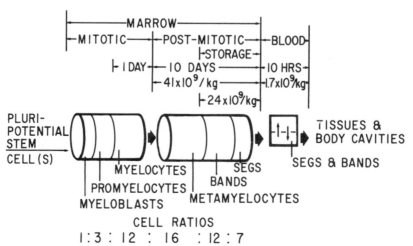

FIGURE 14. Kinetics and overall size of marrow and blood neutrophil pools.

storage pool of bands and segmented neutrophils contains roughly 15 to 20 times as many cells as are in the blood at any time.

There are more segmented neutrophils in the blood than there are bands. (Fig. 15 shows the distinction between bands and segs.) Conversely, in the bone marrow, there are more bands than there are segmented neutrophils. This means that segmented neutrophils are released from the bone marrow to the blood in preference to bands. However, when demand for release of cells from bone marrow to the blood is accelerated, the storage pool of segmented neutrophils is exhausted first and the proportion of bands released steadily increases. This, in turn, is reflected by an increase in the proportion of bands in the blood.

When an increased ratio of bands to segs is found in the blood, with or without an increase in more immature neutrophils such as metamyelocytes, it is indicative of accelerated marrow release, usually accompanied by a reduction in size of the storage pool, and is often referred to as a "shift to the left." The credit for this peculiar phrase must go to those who read and referred to an article by Arneth, published in 1904. He divided blood neutrophils into more than 20 categories and portrayed them from left to right on the page, in order of supposedly increasing maturity; so a "shift to the left" refers to a shift from relatively mature to immature neutrophils in the blood. In more recent years, many laboratory sheets have reported the percentage of neutrophils to the left, other WBC to the right, and "shift to the left" often has been used incorrectly to denote any increase in percentage of any type of neutrophil on the blood smear.

The mechanism by which neutrophils leave the marrow is quite dissimilar from the mechanism by which they subsequently leave the blood. Marrow egress is accomplished by the neutrophil moving *through* the endothelial cells separating marrow parynchyma from a venous sinus (see Fig. 6, top). Diapedesis (egress from the blood) (see page 38) occurs *between* endothelial cells (see Fig. 6, bottom). Movement through the endothelial cell is accompanied by the creation of fenestrations which are not apparent in the absence of cell transit. These pores are smaller in diameter than the traversing cell, so that the traversing cell must be quite pliable to move through them. Erythrocytes (reticulocytes) leave the marrow in the same fashion. Megakaryocytes generally extend a snake-like cytoplasmic process through the pore, sections of which are then severed in the sinus, which then circulate as platelets. Some megakaryocytes

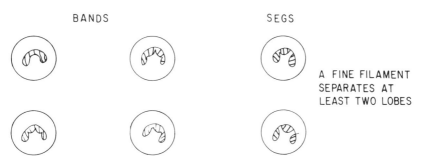

BANDS   SEGS

A FINE FILAMENT SEPARATES AT LEAST TWO LOBES

FIGURE 15. Morphologic distinction between bands and segmented neutrophils.

are released intact, quickly lodging in pulmonary arterioles and breaking up and releasing platelets.

The mechanism by which the neutrophil system is regulated has not been entirely clarified. If neutropenia is produced experimentally in animals or in man, an unidentified hormone appears in plasma which accelerates the rate of release of neutrophils from the bone marrow storage pool to the blood (neutrophil-releasing factor); a different factor is required for growth of colonies of neutrophils in semi-solid media (colony-stimulating factor, CSF). CSF is the primary candidate for a hormone stimulating neutrophil production in the intact animal.

KINETIC CHANGES IN DISEASE

There are three primary factors or combinations of these three factors that influence blood neutrophil concentration: (1) rate of input of neutrophils from the bone marrow storage pool to the blood, (2) proportion of cells that are circulating as compared with marginated in the blood, and (3) rate at which cells are leaving the blood.

In man, severe exercise or administration of epinephrine will decrease the proportion of marginated cells and therefore induce neutrophilia. This pseudo-neutrophilia (so called because there is no change in the total number of neutrophils in the blood) occurs in the absence of any change in input or output. We assume that it explains transient instances of neutrophilia encountered in a variety of clinical situations. For example, a child, terrified by white coats and needles, has neutrophilia in the first blood sample obtained. Later, when the child is a bit blasé about hospital procedures, the blood sample yields normal values. The discrepancy between the two tests necessitates yet a third, which also is normal. One assumes that all values were correct; neutrophilia on the first test reflecting demargination induced by epinephrine. In animals, anesthesia with either ether or pentobarbital induces an increase in the proportion of cells that are marginated, inducing a pseudo-neutropenia. This type of neutropenia may account for numerous instances of neutropenia in man; it accounts for the transient neutropenia that regularly accompanies the onset of hemodialysis, and for that in certain infections such as malaria and certain viral infections. Since neither pseudo-neutrophilia nor pseudo-neutropenia is associated with any increase or decrease in the rate at which cells are entering from the bone marrow, they are not associated with any shift in the proportion of bands to segs in the blood.

Kinetics of neutrophils in *infection* represents a balance between changing rates of outflow from the blood and inflow from the marrow to the blood. The inflammatory stimulus leads to increased margination with very transient pseudo-neutropenia in some instances. Outflow rapidly accelerates, as does inflow. In most infections, inflow accelerates until outflow is exceeded, and an increase in blood neutrophil concentration develops (Figs. 16 and 17).

When the infection is very severe, such a large number of neutrophils may be demanded at the site of infection that the storage pool of the bone marrow is exhausted. This is especially likely to happen in diseases in which the storage

CIRCULATING

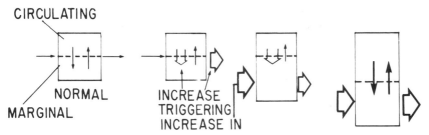

NORMAL
MARGINAL

INCREASE
TRIGGERING
INCREASE IN

FIGURE 16. Blood response to inflammation.

pool is diminished in size (most patients with neutropenia, patients under treatment with cell poisons, in B_{12} and folic acid deficiency, and so forth). Even if cell production increases in response to infection, it cannot keep apace in some instances, and neutropenia develops (see Fig. 17).

Since such a series of events signifies a relative deficit of phagocytes at the site of infection, it is not surprising that development of neutropenia during the course of severe, acute pyogenic infection, such as pneumonococcal pneumonia, is a grave prognostic sign.

If chronic infection develops, neutrophil concentration may remain high and a "new steady state" of balanced but increased neutrophil input and output is maintained by accelerating production. Indeed, most instances of chronic

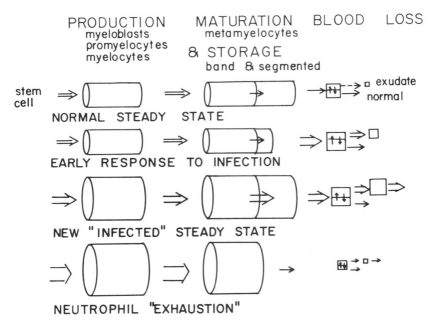

FIGURE 17. Changes in overall patterns of neutrophil kinetics during infection.

neutrophilia (for example, as seen with polycythemia vera or Hodgkin's disease) represent a "new steady state" of blood kinetics. Input and output are equal but abnormally large, and production is increased (see Fig. 17).

Administration of pharmacologic doses of *adrenal glucocorticosteroids* (cortisol or its analogs) induces neutrophilia. In this instance, neutrophilia develops primarily due to decreased output, but is accompanied by a transient increase in input as well as a slight shift from the marginal pool to the circulating pool. This "dam on the stream" results in a seemingly ambiguous phenomenon. The number of cells that will enter an exudate by diapedesis is reduced despite an increase in blood neutrophil concentration. This probably explains, at least in part, why patients receiving steroid therapy are prone to develop serious infections.

Neutropenia thus can be associated with a variety of kinetic changes (Fig. 18), but most commonly is due to decreased production. Decreased production can be the result of many causes (Table 4).

Determining the *ratio of bands to segs* in blood is useful in interpreting changes in neutrophil kinetics. In normal subjects, this ratio varies from less than 0.1 to approximately 0.3. However, day-to-day variation in a given subject is less than the variation between different subjects. In any situation in which output is accelerating, the ratio of bands to segs in blood will increase as the size of the storage pool of the marrow decreases. Bands and segs marginate and leave the blood at approximately equal rates. In any situation in which there is a continuing excessive demand for cells, production will increase as long as the bone marrow is normal; in this case, as the storage pool is reconstituted or even increases in size (see Fig. 17), the band to seg ratio may return to normal.

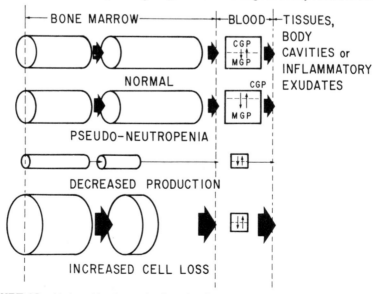

FIGURE 18. Various kinetic mechanisms leading to neutropenia. (Courtesy of Sallie S. Boggs.)

TABLE 4. Examples of Types of Neutropenia*

Kinetic Defect and Its Cause:

Decreased Production
Congenital*
Dominantly inherited—reduced feed-in from stem cells.
Recessively inherited (Kostmann's syndrome)—increased feed-in from stem cells but either cell death or "maturation arrest" beyond the promyelocytic stage.
Cyclic—cyclic variation in feed-in from stem cells, so that blood neutrophils "cycle" from normal to $\pm$ zero levels every 21 days, and other myeloid hematopoietic cells also cycle.
Drug induced
Cytotoxic therapy or accidental exposure—all dividing cells or even resting stem cells may be damaged and/or killed.
Idiosyncratic—an occasional patient develops neutropenia (often severe) due to loss of neutrophil precursors at doses that have no effect in most patients.
Associated with other diseases
Acute leukemias—? leukemic stem cell is recognized by the normal control mechanisms as if it were a normal cell, and stem cell output declines?
Vitamin B_{12} and folate deficiency—number of neutrophil precursors in the marrow is actually increased, but they die in the marrow (ineffective hematopoiesis).

Increased Destruction or Loss of Neutrophils from Blood
Immune mediated
Idiopathic—antineutrophil antibody, IgG usually, coats the neutrophil so that it is phagocytosed by macrophages.
Neonatal (transient)—mother sensitized against fetus neutrophils by previous pregnancy or by receipt of blood products, and her resultant antibodies cross placenta.
Drug induced
hapten type—drug as antigen induces antibody that crossreacts with neutrophils.
"accidental passenger"—antibody is to drug but drug binds to neutrophil so antibody also affects neutrophil.
Associated with other diseases
Felty's syndrome (rheumatoid arthritis with neutropenia and splenomegaly)—antibody develops that may also react with marrow precursors as well as with blood neutrophils so production is highly variable.
Severe pyogenic infection (see text)

Pseudo-Neutropenia—shift from circulating to marginal pool without change in total number of blood neutrophils (see text).

Reduced Release From Marrow—(production and size of the storage pool are normal or increased)
Congenital diseases in which the mature neutrophil seems functionally abnormal, termed "myelokathexis" and "lazy leukocyte syndrome" (the latter has also been reported as an acquired disease).

*This is a very incomplete list; for example, there are at least three varieties of dominantly-inherited neutropenia of variable severity, but all have been associated with decreased production.

Neutropenia is the most common cause of overall neutrophil dysfunction. An absolute neutrophil count of less than 500 cells per µl is a life-threatening condition; patients with this abnormality are highly susceptible to overwhelming bacterial or fungal infections. Furthermore, this risk increases enormously if the total count falls still further. Actually, the level of blood neutrophils in and of itself is a very poor predictor for development of infection. The risk of infection in the presence of neutropenia is increased by many ancillary factors, such as concurrent monocytopenia, thrombocytopenia, immune suppression, and reduced integrity of mucosal surfaces. The most frequent cause of severe neutropenia is cytotoxic drugs, such as those used to treat cancer or leukemia. Autoimmune diseases, aplastic anemia, infiltrative diseases of the marrow, and idiosyncratic reactions to drugs are other important causes of severe neutropenia. The major clinical feature of this condition is the rapidity and overwhelming nature of the associated infection. Patients may present with a low-grade fever without localizing signs. Because of the defect in this host defense mechanism, these individuals may die within 24 hours due to overwhelming sepsis. Thus, fever in a neutropenic patient must be considered a medical emergency.

Neutrophil Function

In order to successfully attack an invading microorganism, the neutrophil must leave the blood, migrate into the area of beginning infection, and then recognize, phagocytize, kill, and digest the invader. We have divided these events into two broad categories, termed the migration cascade and the killing cascade.

THE MIGRATION CASCADE

This overall movement involves closely-related but distinct events (distinct in the sense that somewhat separate mechanisms are involved; closely-related in that some stimuli can initiate more than one event). The migration cascade begins with

Margination of blood neutrophils (see page 34);
but a neutrophil can marginate without actually undergoing Adherence (and Aggregation).

With the process of adherence, the neutrophil attaches to the vascular endothelium and undergoes spreading on its surface. Adherence ordinarily is accompanied by aggregation, although the latter may occur in circulation and adherence of the aggregated neutrophils occurs when they reach a capillary bed (see dialysis-induced neutropenia, page 48). Adherence can be further subdivided on the basis of the strength of attachment into "attachment," a passive, easily reversed process, and "anchoring," an energy-dependent, less easily reversed process. In inflamed areas, adherent neutrophils may become unattached, re-entering freely circulating blood (but without having left vascular confines) or may undergo

Diapedesis.

This process (see Fig. 6) takes place by movement through junctional areas between endothelial cells, followed by a breaking through of the basement membrane, perhaps aided by release of substances such as protease by the migrating neutrophil. Thereafter, the neutrophil will migrate in tissues or in body cavities in two basic ways:

Random migration or

Directed migration (response to a chemotactic stimulus).

Once the neutrophil enters the area of significantly inflamed tissue, it may migrate back out (but not back to blood), die (and be phagocytosed by macrophages in the area), or be

Immobilized but still functionally intact.

The integrity of the entire migration cascade is tested *in vivo* by inducing an inflammation and measuring the number of neutrophils that enter an exudate. In man, this usually is done with the "skin window" technique. A small area of skin is superficially abraded and then covered with a glass coverslip. The coverslip is removed periodically and stained as if it were a blood smear. Normally, within an hour, a few neutrophils have migrated in and adhered to the glass; by 6 hours a fairly uniform monolayer of neutrophils is present, corresponding to the area of the abrasion. By 24 hours, approximately half of the cells on the glass are monocytes. Alternatively, the abrasion can be covered with a chamber filled with autologous serum and the total number of neutrophils migrating into the chamber can be quantified ($>25 \times 10^6$ neutrophils should enter a 1-ml chamber within 24 hours). A reduced cellular response in a skin window, in the absence of neutropenia, indicates an abnormality at one or more points in the above migration cascade.

The overall integrity of the cascade also can be tested *in vitro,* although this testing might miss defects in migration and/or endothelial adherence. For example, a "Boyden chamber" is a closed system with two sides separated by a filter; the holes in the filter are smaller than neutrophils, but large enough (0.45 μm) to allow cells to deform and migrate from one side to the other. Neutrophils are placed in one side and a chemotactic stimulus is placed in the other. With a normal response, more neutrophils are found on and in the filter on the side to which the chemotactic stimulus was added than on the side to which the neutrophils were exposed initially.

If an abnormality is detected in either (or both) of these "screening" tests, the more exact site of the defect in the cascade and whether the defect resides in the neutrophil or in generation of a necessary extraneutrophil influence is explored.

CHEMOTAXINS. These are naturally occurring or synthetic substances. When a cell capable of directed migration is exposed to a chemical gradient of a chemotaxin for which that cell has a receptor, the cell moves in the direction of highest chemical concentration. There is a wide variety of naturally occurring chemotaxins that are released or are generated as part of inflammatory reactions. These include cleavage fragments generated by activation of complement such as C5a and C5a-des-arginine; secretion products of activated mast cells, lymphocytes, monocyte-macrophages, and the neutrophil itself; proteins generated from coagulation and kinin pathway activation, and products of invading bacteria and viruses. Metabolites from lipo-oxygenation of arachidonic acid are particularly potent chemotaxins for neutrophils, especially one termed leukotriene B. It is generally assumed that *all* of these (and others) play specific roles *in vivo,* but proof for an *in vivo* role for most chemotaxins is lacking. Synthetic, and presumably not naturally occurring, chemotaxins are frequently employed in *in vivo* or *in vitro* experimental studies; principally the formylmethionine molecule, N-fMet-Leu-Phe (fMLP). fMLP is closely related in structure to certain bacterially derived chemotaxins. Similar to certain natural chemotaxins, such as leukotriene B and C5a, it primarily attracts neutrophils, but also attracts other cells to a lesser degree.

The normal human neutrophil has approximately 50,000 receptors for fMLP. Binding of fMLP to a receptor (or of other chemotaxins such as C5a to other, distinct receptors) initiates a very complex series of poorly-defined chemical events that result in a polarized contraction of the cell associated with reorganization of such cytoskeletal elements as microfilaments and microtubules. Such a cell is *"oriented"* (Fig. 19). The first detectable change following binding of a chemotaxin to a neutrophil plasma membrane receptor is membrane hyperpolarization. Ion flux accelerates, especially that of calcium. Other metabolic changes include alterations in synthesis and turnover of methylated phospholipids, changes in cAMP and cGMP, and activation of phospholipase which releases arachi-

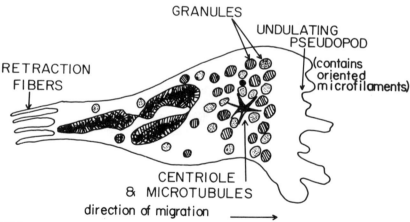

FIGURE 19. An "oriented" neutrophil. In response to a chemotactic stimulus, the neutrophil becomes oriented and moves toward the higher concentration area of the chemotaxin gradient. At the leading edge of the cell is an undulating pseudopod (termed a lamellaepodia) that is rich in actin- and myosin-containing microfilaments. Most granules are between the undulating pseudopod and the nucleus. The nucleus moves toward the rear of the cell, trailed by long "retraction fibers." Eosinophils assume a virtually identical orientation appearance to that of neutrophils, but monocytes do so to a lesser extent. (Courtesy of Sallie S. Boggs.)

donic acid, generating prostaglandins and leukotrienes. Locomotion may be mediated by actin-myosin contractile proteins and the cell contents are oriented and stabilized by microtubules directed from the centriole. Neutrophils crawl but do not swim; thus, a surface is required for their locomotion. Orientation and locomotion can be separated in *in vitro* test systems. Low levels of magnesium in the suspending media are required for locomotion but not for orientation. Locomotion in the form of random migration occurs without orientation; such cells will wander about on a surface to which they are only loosely adherent. In the presence of a chemotactic factor, but in the absence of a gradient (that is, the factor is uniformly distributed throughout the media suspending the neutrophil), orientation occurs, but movement is random. However, random movement in the presence of a chemotactic factor is more active, and attachment is firmer than in its absence ("chemokinesis").

The oriented neutrophil is very sensitive to chemotaxins and when presented with as small a gradient as 1 percent from head to tail, moves in a directional fashion. Its continued migration must involve repeated release of attached surfaces and reattachment. Continued recognition of a gradient may involve generation of new receptors at the leading edge of the cell with posterior movement and loss or inactivation of occupied receptors. However, within a relatively brief time, the neutrophil becomes refractory to chemotactic stimuli (becomes "tolerant") and is relatively immobile. This refractoriness is not well understood but probably is multifactorial. The chemotaxins themselves are deactivated by a variety of products generated in the inflammatory response, including an inhibitor released from neutrophil granules.

Neutrophil aggregation and adhesion are promoted by chemotactic stimuli, but the actual process may be initiated by a cleavage product of C5a and also by other substances such as thromboxanes and endogenous pyrogen. Also stimulated are certain events in the "killing cascade" (see below), such as oxidative metabolism, increase in the number of complement receptors, and degranulation.

THE KILLING CASCADE

Once the neutrophil enters the vicinity of the foreign invader via the migration cascade, the killing cascade is initiated. Actually, as with virtually all neutrophil functions, a neat separation of activities is not present. For example, chemotactic stimulation has some initiating effects on events that we have listed in the killing cascade, such as degranulation. During migration, some secondary granules fuse with the undulating pseudopod, releasing contents such as collagenase which may aid the cell in moving through tissues.

The process of killing begins virtually simultaneously with the process of phagocytosis. While we ordinarily consider killing by phagocytes to be synonymous with endocytosis, this is not always the case. Large objects can be attacked and killed without complete endocytosis (see eosinophils, page 54).

The killing cascade begins with

Recognition

of the invader and
Attachment
of the neutrophil to the invader.

These are closely-linked events involving specific receptors. For example, if a bacteria has been attacked by immunoglobulin (Ig) or has complement bound to its surface, it is attached to the neutrophil via receptors for the Fc region of Ig and/or C3b receptors.

Once recognition has been followed by attachment, the next series of events occurs or begins virtually at the same time. However, there is evidence to suggest that these are separately regulated, at least in part. For example, treatment of cells with cytochalasin B can separately influence phagocytosis, granule release, and the oxidative burst.

Phagocytosis
begins with pseudopods protruding and surrounding the bacterium. This membrane movement is thought to be initiated and performed via the actin-myosin microfilaments, which also were given credit for the cell's crawling motion (see discussion above). When the leading edge of two pseudopods surrounding the bacterium touch, they fuse. By this fusion mechanism, the bacterium is internalized within a *phagosome* (Fig. 20). The phagosome was initially the cytoplasmic membrane but it is "inside out."

Lysosomal (granule) fusion
involves fusion of granules with each other, with the cytoplasmic membrane in the area of bacterial attachment, and with the phagosome's membrane. Under ordinary circumstances, granules remain separated from one another and from the plasma membrane. Fusion involves a stripping of microfilaments from the plasma membrane and numerous chemical changes in membranes. This fusion with resultant expulsion of granule contents extracellularly or into the phagosome is called

Degranulation.

The granules of neutrophils are of two types, primary (azurophilic) and secondary (specific) (see page 4). There are similarities and differences in the behavior and chemical composition of the two types of granules. For example, both are involved in the process of granule-phagosome fusion but only specific granules are involved in exocytosis, in which their contents are released by fusion of the granule with the cytoplasmic membrane during the migration cascade. Certain enzyme contents, such as lysozyme, are shared by both types of granules, but peroxidase and acid phosphatase are limited to primary granules, and alkaline phosphatase to secondary granules. Actual killing of ingested organisms is not a major, direct effect of granule contents (see discussion below). Most of the granule enzymes are more involved in digestion of already killed organisms than in killing them.

Coincident with phagocytosis, respiration accelerates markedly although some increase in activity is associated with the migration cascade. This is commonly referred to as the

Respiratory burst
and results in the generation of oxidants, as killing compounds, derived

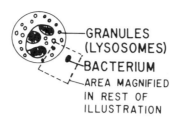

GRANULES
(LYSOSOMES)
BACTERIUM
AREA MAGNIFIED
IN REST OF
ILLUSTRATION

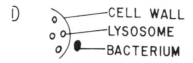

1)
CELL WALL
LYSOSOME
BACTERIUM

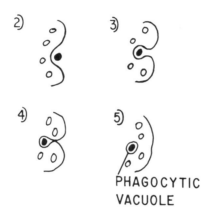

2)   3)

4)   5)

PHAGOCYTIC
VACUOLE

FIGURE 20. The physical process of phagocytosis.

from partial oxygen reduction primarily via the hexose-monophosphate shunt. Many substances will activate the respiratory burst, and activation is energy dependent and reversible but it does not require either ingestion or degranulation. A membrane-bound oxidase is activated; NADPH is a prime candidate as its substrate but NADH also may serve as substrate. This oxidase catalyzes the reaction:

$$2O_2 + NADPH \rightarrow 2O_2^- + NADP$$

Hydrogen peroxide is in turn generated from the superoxide (O_2^-):

$$2O_2^- + 2H^+ \xrightarrow[\text{or superoxide dismutase}]{\text{spontaneous}} H_2O_2 + O_2$$

HMP shunt activity is stimulated by increased NADP availability via the first reaction (above) and by H_2O_2 detoxification:

$$2GSH + H_2O_2 \xrightarrow{\text{glutathione peroxidase}} GSSG + H_2O$$

$$GSSG + NADPH \xrightarrow{\text{glutathione reductase}} 2GSH + NADP$$

These early biochemical events can be thought of as O_2^- production, followed by H_2O_2 production, as a consequence of HMPS activation.

O$_2$-dependent killing is postulated to involve what has been termed the peroxide-hallide (Cl^-)-myeloperoxidase mechanism and formation of highly reactive oxidizing radicals:

$$H_2O_2 + Cl^- \xrightarrow{\text{myeloperoxidase}} HOCl + H_2O$$

and

$$H_2O_2 + O_2^- \; (+/- \text{ other peroxide compounds}) \xrightarrow{\text{iron}} \text{hydroxyl radical} + ?$$

The exact mechanism by which oxidizing radicals kill microorganisms is unknown. Superoxide itself is not a killer but evanescently present singlet oxygen may be. H_2O_2 alone has a slight killing effect.

Anaerobic killing mechanisms also exist but these are not well characterized, probably because defects in the system have not yet been blamed for human disease. The microenvironment of the phagosome is quite acid and this pH change kills or aids in the killing of some organisms (pneumococci). A few of the enzymes in granules are also capable of microbicidal reactions; these include lysozyme in both granules, arginase and glucosidase in primary granules, and lactoferrin in secondary granules. Certain of the cationic granular proteins (positively-charged at physiologic pH) can kill. One such protein which is an efficient killer of *E. coli* and certain other Gram-negative (but not Gram-positive) bacteria has been purified.

Pathogens are not all killed by the same biochemical mechanisms, which explains, in part, why specific defects may be associated with specific types of infection (see page 00).

Finally, the killed microorganism within the phagosome is
digested
by various granule constituents, and the phagosome may be
exocytosed
thus cleansing the cell of its debris. Actually, in the case of neutrophils, digestion and exocytosis do not seem to be very important events (although they are for monocyte-macrophages, as discussed later in this chapter). Most

neutrophils apparently die after a short time in exudates, and in turn are phagocytosed and digested by macrophages.

The *killing capacity* of neutrophils for bacteria, as studied *in vitro*, is considerable but not unlimited. More than 30 pseudomonas organisms can be ingested by individual neutrophils but only about 20 can be killed. One might say that appetite overestimates digestive capacity. As the ratio of bacteria to neutrophils is increased, the average number of bacteria killed per neutrophil is increased, but the percentage of total bacteria killed is decreased. In other words, the higher the number of bacteria in an infection, the greater the number of neutrophils required to clear them.

Self-regulation of the neutrophil's inflammatory response can occur at many points in the two cascades; that is, products formed or released by the neutrophil during its activation in inflammation in turn modulate its activation. For example, the "killing complex," myeloperoxidase-H_2O_2-hallide, inactivates the chemotactic effect of C5a. The complete complex is more active than its parts because myeloperoxidase-hallide is less effective and H_2O_2 is ineffective.

DEFECTS IN THE FUNCTIONAL CASCADES
OF MIGRATION AND KILLING

There is a long and growing list of congenital and acquired diseases associated with abnormalities of neutrophil function, almost all of which are "new" diseases. Defects can be roughly divided into defects residing in the neutrophil or defects in mediators of neutrophil function. For each of these, both congenital and acquired types of defects have been described.

Chronic granulomatous disease (CGD) can be considered the index disease involving congenitally defective neutrophils. This relatively rare, sex-linked, inherited disorder was described as a clinical entity in the 1950s. It is almost uniformly fatal in childhood, and the affected boys suffer from chronic, granulomatous infections with bacteria ordinarily considered to be of low-grade pathogenicity, such as enterobacteriacae, serratia, and coagulase-negative staphylococci. Evaluation of their immune systems had indicated them to be normal and their neutrophils were of normal number and appeared to respond normally to infection. However, in 1966, Holmes and co-workers reported that while CGD neutrophils phagocytosed bacteria, they failed to kill them. The defect in CGD is in activation of the membrane oxidase that initiates the respiratory burst (see page 43). Thus, H_2O_2 is not generated and is missing from the normal H_2O_2-hallide-myeloperoxidase killing complex. Catalase-positive organisms are phagocytosed, but not killed. Catalase-negative bacteria, such as pneumococci and β-hemolytic streptococci, produce H_2O_2 and thus engineer their own demise. Eosinophils and monocytes also are affected by the abnormality. Several patients with defects in killing closely related to that of CGD have been described, some of whom were girls.

Complement deficiency presents a defect extrinsic to the phagocyte which also is associated with an increase in pyogenic infection in certain types of deficiency. Congenital C3 deficiency directly influences phagocytosis and inter-feres with generation of other components important for chemotaxis, such as C5a. Deficiencies of C1r, C2, and C4 have been associated with abnormal neutrophil responses measured *in vitro,* but not with increased infection. Presumably, the alternate pathway of activation (Fig. 21) is sufficient to bypass these defects *in vivo.*

Certain of the many other defects in neutrophil function are mentioned in Table 5, but the list is in no sense all-inclusive. Some, such as CGD, routinely lead to death from infection, while others, such as acatalasemia, are not asso-ciated with any increase in infectious problems. Absence of infection in the presence of a neutrophil defect presumably reflects the alternative and overlap-ping pathways available to contain and kill invading organisms.

ADVERSE EFFECTS OF NEUTROPHILS

Adverse consequences can result from inflammatory reactions and from the neutrophil's participation in them. The effect of neutrophil products upon various tissues and constituents of tissues can be easily documented, but documenta-tion of the importance of this as a causative factor in human disease is more difficult. Two examples will be given. There is fairly good evidence that the neutrophil plays a major role in the pathogenesis of the actual *gouty attack.*

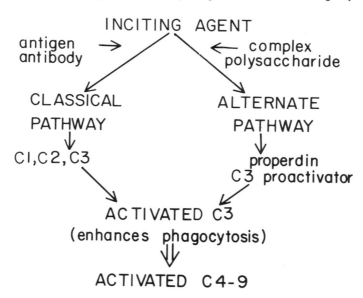

FIGURE 21. Mechanism of activating chemotactic components of complement. (Cour-tesy of Sallie S. Boggs.)

TABLE 5. Examples of Defects Involving Neutrophil Function

Defects in the Migration Cascade
  Congenital complement deficiency (see text)
  Generation of chemotactic factors
    Is inhibited in uremia, and congenital absence of chemotactic lymphokines has been
    described.
  Acquired production of chemotactic inhibitors
    In cancer, renal dialysis, chronic infections, and so forth, as well as idiopathic (?
    usually an IgG).
  Congenital absence of a membrane glycoprotein
    Defective attachment, absent migration, associated with marked neutrophilia and
    increased neutrophil production, but with severe, recurrent infection.
  "Job's" syndrome
    Defective chemotactic response with "boils" (also increased IgE, eosinophilia, eczema).
    Levamisole seems to restore chemotaxis to normal, but does not improve recurrent
    boils.
  "Lazy leukocyte" syndrome
    The neutrophil defect (undefined) that leads to neutropenia (reduced release from
    marrow) also is associated with reduced adhesion and migration.

Defects in the Killing Cascade
  Chronic granulomatous disease (see text)
  Glucose-6-phosphate dehydrogenase deficiency
    If severe, there is inefficient NADPH generation with a killing defect and infectious
    problems.
  Myeloperoxidase deficiency
    Minimal problems, mostly with *Candida* infections. Alternate means of generating
    oxidizing radicals are generally sufficient for killing.
  Deficiency of H_2O_2 detoxifying enzymes
    Detectable changes in duration of killing-associated events, but not associated with
    increased frequency of infection (glutathione reductase, catalase, dismutase).

Defects with Significant Influence on Both Cascades
  Congenital absence of specific granules
    Adherence and aggregation were supranormal, and chemotaxis, killing, and respira-
    tory burst were decreased in a patient with severe infection.
  Congenital absence of actin polymerization
    Cells can adhere, but adherence is not stimulated by chemotaxins, and migration
    and phagocytosis are inhibited.
  Defects in microtubule assembly
    Congenital increase in assembly with increased infection, defective orientation,
    chemotaxis and phagocytosis.
    Decreased assembly is seen with the Chediak-Higashi syndrome (see text).
    Various drugs (such as vincristine, vinblastine, colchicine) poison microtubules.
  Diabetes and other causes of hyperosmolality
    Virtually all neutrophil responses are sluggish but return to normal when severe
    hyperglycemia is corrected.
  Alcohol intoxication
    Virtually all neutrophil responses are sluggish but are corrected quickly when the cell
    "sobers up," secondary to the patient doing the same.

Gout itself, of course, is precipitated by excessive uric acid. However, the formation of urate crystals in joint fluid attracts neutrophils, the forming exudate acidifies joint fluid, thus precipitating more crystal formation, more inflammation, and so forth. Colchicine, which in adequate doses will abort an acute attack of gout, does so by paralyzing neutrophils through poisoning their microtubules. *Hemodialysis,* most commonly used for the treatment of renal failure, results in a highly predictable sequence of events that can be summarized as follows. Initial contact of the patient's plasma with the cellophane membrane of the dialysis apparatus results in complement activation. The $C5a_{desarginine}$ fragment induces aggregation of neutrophils in blood leaving the apparatus, and these aggregates lodge in capillaries or precapillary vessels in the lungs. Since adhesion as well as aggregation is enhanced by $C5a_{desarginine}$, initial adherence of the leukocytes is quite firm, and secondary granule products may be released. Neutrophil-neutral proteases can degrade elastin, collagen, proteoglycans, and basement membrane. However, their potential damaging effect can be modulated by a local pulmonary antiprotease (which is inactivated by cigarette smoke). Since metabolic activities of these aggregated, adherent neutrophils are activated, superoxide and hydroxyl radicals may also be released as potentially damaging agents, but these may also inactivate granule enzymes before or during their release from the cell. In addition, mechanical blockade induces a sudden increase in pulmonary artery pressure that may induce respiratory distress in patients with underlying pulmonary and/or cardiac disease. Within a few minutes, the neutrophil becomes "down regulated," is refractory to $C5a_{desarginine}$, and deaggregation occurs. These events are reflected in sudden and fairly profound neutropenia which develops during the first 15 minutes of the dialysis procedure. Neutropenia is then quickly reversed and, as extra marrow release is stimulated, an "overshoot" neutrophilia follows.

Morphologic Abnormalities of Neutrophils

These usually are not evident in the above diseases. However, there are a variety of congenital and acquired diseases (or at least abnormalities) that can be detected by examining neutrophils in a blood smear. We will discuss only two of these.

The *Chediak-Higashi syndrome* is a very rare syndrome characterized by giant granules in neutrophils (and in monocytes, eosinophils, mast cells, basophils, osteoclasts, and so forth, all products of the HSC). The disease is inherited as an autosomal recessive and is of fairly major interest to investigators since it occurs in many species in addition to man (e.g., mouse, cow, mink, killer whale). Death from infection is common. Abnormally large (but sparse) azurophilic granules characterize the disease but, as such, may play a minimal role in the disease's defect in neutrophil function. There is defective assembly of microtubules so that many portions of both the migration and killing cascades are affected. If cellular cGMP is increased or if cAMP is decreased, defective neutrophil function is improved or corrected. Oculocutaneous albinism and abnormal bleeding are also a part of the syndrome, the bleeding probably reflecting a platelet defect. The platelets have decreased serotonin and decreased "dense bodies," the storage organelle for serotonin. If normal platelets (or serotonin) are added *in vitro* or *in vivo* to Chediak-Higashi neutrophils, the neutrophil killing defect is corrected. This observation strengthens the case for there being potentially important functional interactions of platelets and phagocytes.

The *Pelger-Huët anomaly* is characterized by reduced segmentation of neutrophils. It is reasonably common; the heterozygous form occurs in approximately 1 in 5,000 persons. Neutrophils contain no nuclear lobes or two (occasionally three) lobes, but the chromatin is quite dense so they do not appear as band neutrophils. In the homozygous form, no lobes are present; the neutrophil has an oval nucleus but with "mature" chromatin structure. However, these neutrophils appear to function in a nearly normal fashion and there is, at most, a questionable increase in the frequency of infection. *Acquired* forms of Pelger-Huët-like cells are seen in patients with AML and related diseases.

MONOCYTES AND MACROPHAGES

This is the "oldest" cell in the hematopoietic systems; for example, the limulus (horseshoe crab), an animal unchanged for millions of years, has but a single type of cell in its blood, an "amoebocyte" which bears some resemblance to mammalian macrophages.

Terminology, as developed in medicine (or in other fields), often is tortuous in derivation, confusing, and inexact. This problem, as it relates specifically to hematology, is particularly evident with respect to the monocyte-macrophage system. Blood monocytes have often been "lumped" with lymphocytes as "blood mononuclear cells," presumably, as opposed to "polymorphonuclear." Perhaps that usage has led to the current popularity of "mononuclear phagocyte system (or complex)" as a term encompassing monocytes and macrophages. However, macrophages are one of the few normal cells that may be truly multinuclear (polyploid) (see discussion below), and there certainly are numerous other types of cells that are mononuclear and capable of phagocytosis. "Reticuloendothelial system" once was the most popular term used to encompass the monocyte-macrophage system and still is in fairly widespread use.

BLOOD MONOCYTES. These are immature cells that are produced in marrow and migrate into tissues and body cavities where they mature into so-called "fixed" and "wandering" macrophages (pulmonary-alveolar macrophages, pleural and peritoneal cavity macrophages, macrophages lining sinuses, and also located elsewhere in spleen and marrow, Kupfer cells in liver, Langerhan's cells in epidermis, and so forth).

Monocytes share a terminal or nearly terminal stem cell with neutrophils (see Figs. 2 and 3) following which their maturation pathways diverge. However, pro-monocytes are quite similar in appearance to pro-myelocytes in ordinary preparations of bone marrow. In fact, immature monocytes usually are not recognized as such and are enumerated with neutrophil precursors in differential counts of normal bone marrow. This small (relative to neutrophils) population can be detected if marrow smears are stained for certain forms of esterases. Following two to three doubling divisions in the post-stem cell marrow production (and maturation) pool, monocytes are released to the blood. Unlike the neutrophil, there is no appreciable storage pool of monocytes in marrow.

The blood transit time is fairly rapid, averaging approximately 14 hours (as compared with 10 for the neutrophil). Like the neutrophil, it leaves the blood in a random fashion, exit being independent of time of entry from the bone marrow.

MATURATION INTO MACROPHAGES. The site of lodgement of the monocyte seems to influence the nature of maturation. For example, the enzymatic composition of pulmonary and peritoneal macrophages is not identical. As might be expected, pulmonary macrophages are more active in an aerobic environment, whereas peritoneal cells function better in anaerobic conditions. Maturation involves synthesis of new or more enzymes, increased endoplasmic reticulum, and probably synthesis of more granules. At the same time, certain enzymes (peroxidase) are lost from granules as monocytes mature into macrophages. Macrophages may fuse with one another resulting in large, polyploid cells. Langerhan's giant cell, found in granulomatous inflammation, such as that produced by tuberculosis, is the classic example, but polyploid macrophages occur in the absence of any evident inflammatory stimulus. Normally, tissue macrophages have a long (but not carefully measured) life-span. Presumably, the blood monocyte turnover rate, approximately $\frac{1}{20}$th that for neutrophils, reflects the number of macrophages replaced each day. However, the total mass of macrophages has not been measured. A demand for an accelerated rate of replacement of tissue macrophages can stimulate replication of an *in situ* cell (presumably the macrophage itself) as well as attract an accelerated influx of new monocytes; that is, the macrophage, like the lymphocyte, may be capable of acting as its own stem cell. With an inflammatory stimulus, monocytes migrate from blood to the developing exudate but do so at an initially slower rate than neutrophils. Conversely, they eventually far outnumber neutrophils in the inflamed area, particularly as inflammation is resolving (or becoming "granulomatous").

Monocyte-Macrophage Function

The monocyte-macrophage system plays a vital role in multiple host-defense mechanisms. Functions can be broadly grouped into six categories:

1. initiating immune responses
2. regulating the magnitude of immune response
3. phagocytosing and killing microorganisms
4. exerting antitumor activities
5. phagocytosing and degrading effete cells, cellular debris, and other particulate matter
6. secreting various soluble, biologically active substances.

Many of these activities are intimately tied to the functions of T lymphocytes; hence, it is impossible to appreciate the biologic activities of macrophages without understanding the material presented in the lymphocyte section.

In immunologic reactions, macrophages act to process (degrade and chemically modify) antigens and present these immunogens to potentially responsive T and B lymphocytes. Thus, this function serves to initiate both cell-mediated and humoral immune responses. This presentation function greatly enhances the antigenicity of foreign substances; immunogens presented by macrophages are several thousand times more potent than those that are in a soluble form. In subserving this function, only a small number of macrophages is required. Antigenic presentation by macrophages is genetically restricted in that both the macrophage and the responsive lymphocytes must share histo-compatability determinants in order to effect a response.

A second and related immunologic function subserved by macrophages is the release of a soluble factor, interleukin-1 (IL-1) which stimulates T lympho-cytes to elaborate an important growth factor (T cell growth factor [TCGF]), also called interleukin-2 (IL-2). The latter, in turn, serves to promote the proliferative expansion of responsive T cells.

Conversely, macrophages can also act to regulate or suppress certain immune responses. In part, this activity has been attributed to the release of prostaglandins (particularly PGE_2); these arachidonic metabolites have an important influence in inhibiting the immunologic functions of activated lympho-cytes. Excess macrophage inhibition has been implicated as one mechanism involved in several acquired immune deficiency states including the depressed cellular immunity that accompanies Hodgkin's disease (see page 95), chronic disseminated infections, wide-spread malignancies and in patients who have been extensively traumatized.

Macrophages ingest and kill microorganisms by processes quite similar, but not identical, to those discussed for neutrophils. These cells are primarily responsible for destroying or inhibiting the growth of intracellular organisms; these include many relatively resistant pathogens such as mycobacteria, proto-zoa, fungi, viruses, and certain helminths. A key feature of macrophage killing is *cellular activation*. Soluble products of T cells (lymphokines) and a variety of factors, such as interferon, act to alter the metabolic states of resting macro-phages. This process greatly enhances the cell's ability to act as an effector (e.g., kill intracellular organisms, exert antitumor activities). Morphologically, activated macrophages are larger than resting cells and have a greater number of cytoplasmic granules. Functional studies indicate that these activated cells have enhanced abilities to phagocytize particles. One of the major biochemical characteristics of activated cells is increased metabolism of glucose via the hexose-monophosphate shunt.

An *in vivo* murine model useful for understanding the interrelationship between T cells and monocytes involves the killing of the intracellular bacteria, *Listeria monocytogenes*. These bacteria will colonize and persist in resting macrophages. However, if these infected cells are cultured with a soluble product prepared by incubating listeria antigens with T lymphocytes programmed to respond to these antigens, the macrophages become activated and, in turn, rapidly and completely kill the intracellular microorganisms. Macrophage activation and the resultant microbial killing is a nonspecific response. The soluble products elicited by listeria-sensitized T cells and listeria antigens induce a killing reaction in resting macrophages infected with BCG microorganisms as well as listeria.

These data *in toto* suggest a complex interrelationship between macrophages and T lymphocytes. In an appropriate infection, macrophages process microbial antigens and present them to T cells. The T cells, in turn, respond immunologically—they elaborate lymphokines which recruit (chemotaxins) and activate (activating factor) resting macrophages. The latter cells become activated, exert a microbicidal reaction and, at the same time, serve to suppress or turn off the T-cell reaction.

Activated macrophages not only have microbicidal properties, but also are capable of killing several types of cultured tumor cells. This may also be an important *in vivo* function of these cells. Killing appears to be due to a direct cytolytic effect of activated cells, requiring intimate contact but independent of immune (e.g., antigen-specific) activities. Many neoplasms are infiltrated by macrophages and there is suggestive evidence that they exert a protective function. For example, there is a good correlation between the macrophage content of a tumor and survival. One of the goals of the immunotherapeutic protocols used to treat cancer is to boost macrophage tumor cytotoxicity. Macrophages are also capable of lysing tumor cells by an antibody-dependent cellular cytotoxic (ADCC) mechanism, similar to that described for lymphocytes (see page 76). This cytotoxic reaction depends upon an initial attachment of immunoglobulins to the tumor cell. Macrophages then bind to the Ig through Fc receptors and exert a lytic injury to the tumor cell.

Macrophages have an important role in eliminating effete cells, cellular debris and particulate matter, including activated clotting factors, denatured proteins, and antigen-antibody complexes. This function is subserved by both mobile and fixed phagocytes. For example, in inflammatory exudates, macrophages infiltrate the site and clean up the debris resulting from neutrophil infiltration and destruction of invading microorganisms. Macrophage-like cells lining vascular channels (the reticuloendothelial system) play an essential role in removing potentially toxic substances from the blood. These cells phagocytize such particulates as blood-borne bacteria, activated clotting factors, and antigen-antibody complexes. In addition, they serve to remove dying blood cells, such as aged red cells. This process conserves essential components of the cell—for example, the iron contained in hemoglobin is released and returned to the body's iron pools. Thus, it is available for synthesis of new hemoglobin. It should be noted that in many severe diseases and after extensive trauma, there is a failure of the reticuloendothelial system's clearing functions. This deficit is believed to permit the build-up of potentially toxic material in the circulation. The particulates can promote injuries in multiple organs such as the lungs. The syndrome of multiple organ failure is often the immediate cause of death.

Pathologically, the reticuloendothelial system is responsible for the removal of antibody-coated blood cells. Thus, in syndromes such as autoimmune hemolytic anemia, the patient's own red cells are coated with an autoantibody. These cells are prematurely removed from the circulation and destroyed by the fixed phagocyte. Similar processes have been described in immune-type thrombocytopenia (ITP) in which platelet autoantibodies result in premature sequestration and destruction of these clotting factors.

The macrophage also is an important secretory cell. As previously noted, these cells elaborate IL-1, important in inducing T-cell proliferation, and prostaglandins, important mediators of inflammation. In addition, macrophages elaborate other biologically active substances, including complement components, those effecting platelet activation, and the clotting systems and various proteases that serve to promote degradation of products of inflammation. Macrophages are also a major source of colony-stimulating factor (CSF), a presumed granulocytopoietic hormone, and interferon, a potent antiviral compound.

Diseases of the Monocyte-Macrophage System

Many of the diseases that affect neutrophil function also affect monocyte function. For example, the oxidase defect of chronic granulomatous disease neutrophils (see page 45) is shared by monocytes. However, even though neutrophils and monocytes share a terminal type HSC (see Figs. 2 and 3), production of the two is controlled separately (at least in part). For example, in one form of severe, congenital, dominantly-inherited neutropenia, the marrow contains increased *in vitro* colony-forming cells, but only colonies of monocyte-macrophages are formed. These patients have very few blood neutrophils, but a striking degree of monocytosis. Presumably because of the latter, they have little problem with infection. As one would anticipate, the clonal neoplasms of the myeloid HSC system (see page 15) involve the monocyte. Thus, acute monocytic and "myelomonocytic" leukemia are fairly common morphologic forms of AML (see page 20).

"Histiocyte," is properly used as a synonym for macrophage; that is, most "histiocytes" seen in normal tissue are macrophages. "Reticulum cells," a term happily falling into disuse, included macrophages of normal tissue. However, a common form of lymphoma, currently often referred to as "histiocytic lymphoma" and in the past referred to as "reticulum cell sarcoma," is, in fact, almost always a tumor of B-type lymphocytes, not of monocyte-macrophages.

There are, however, neoplasms primarily involving the monocyte-macrophage system, some of which are malignant. We have placed Hodgkin's disease in that category. Of variable malignancy are the group of syndromes termed "histiocytosis X," including Letterer-Siwe disease, Hand-Schuller-Christian disease, and eosinophilic granuloma. All but the last, which is almost always benign, are seen only in infants and young children. The rare, but uniformly fatal macrophage tumor known as "histiocytic medullary reticulosis" is characterized by an infiltration of large macrophages that actively phagocytose normal red cells and neutrophils.

Gaucher's disease is a "tumor" of macrophages but is not a clonal neoplasm. Rather, it is due to a hereditary deficiency of glucocerebrosidase in macrophage lysosomes and, consequently, has been classed as a "lysosomal storage disease" (along with Nieman-Pick disease, and so forth). The macrophage engulfs effete blood cells but cannot fully digest them, and cerebroside accumulates in the macrophage. A steady and excessive accumulation of large macrophages ensues, producing such findings as massive enlargement of the spleen. Cells similar to Gaucher's cell are seen in such conditions as CML and are the result of delivery of a markedly excessive amount of cerebroside (and other cell products) to the macrophage.

EOSINOPHILS

The colorful appearance of these leukocytes in Romanofsky-stained blood smears has led to a vast amount of literature concerning them, but it is only in the past few years that we have begun to understand their role in host defense. Their overall configuration and the configuration of their marrow precursor compartments are very similar to those of neutrophils, but the similarity pretty much ends there. The two have distinct terminal stem cells as well as distinctively different chemistries, kinetics, and functions. Colonies of eosinophils can be stimulated to grow independently of colonies of neutrophils-macrophages by the action of a specific CSF. This CSF is produced by activated T lymphocytes (and perhaps by other cells), and there is *in vivo* evidence that increased eosinophil production in helminthic infection is mediated by T cells.

The blood transit time of the eosinophil is approximately twice as long as that of the neutrophil, and, unlike the neutrophil, the eosinophil probably returns from tissue to blood and from blood to marrow in normal conditions. Both types of cells can respond to certain of the same *in vivo* inflammatory-chemotactic stimuli, but also to stimuli affecting one cell much more than the other. Unlike neutrophils, many eosinophils normally are found in a nonmyeloid "tissue pool." Scattered eosinophils are found just below epithelial surfaces where these are exposed or potentially exposed to the external environment, such as skin, lungs, gut, lower urinary tract, uterus, and so forth.

Eosinophilia (more than 700 per mm^3, see Table 1) is seen most often in association with infection with metazoic parasites, a variety of allergic conditions, drug hypersensitivity reaction, leukemia-like illnesses, secondary to cancer, or for no discernible reason. As consulting hematologists, we are often asked to see patients because of "eosinophilia." In many circumstances, these consultations are unnecessary, as there is not an absolute increase in these cells. For example, if the leukocyte count is 5000 per mm^3 and eosinophils are reported at 10 percent of the white cell differential, then the absolute count is 500 eosinophils per mm^3, a figure well within the 95 percent confidence limits of normal.

Much more common than eosinophilia is *eosinopenia*. As pointed out in Table 1, normal detection methods exclude the possibility of eosinopenia since 95 percent confidence limits encompass zero. However, failing to easily find eosinophils when a blood smear is "scanned" with 100× magnification is abnormal and indicative of eosinopenia. Absence of eosinophils on repeated examination of blood, marrow, and other tissues has been reported in two patients with allergic phenomena and was thought possibly to be congenital, but absence or scarcity of eosinophils ordinarily reflects a very acute "stressful" situation or an ongoing inflammatory process at the time the blood sample is obtained.

If adrenal glucocorticosteroids are given in pharmacologic doses, blood eosinophils decrease dramatically within two hours. This eosinopenia is due to cell redistribution, not to cell destruction. If steroids are continued, eosinophil levels return to or near to normal within three to four days. Patients with Cushing's disease are *not* eosinopenic. This eosinopenic effect of steroids is thought to explain the eosinopenia that accompanies a wide variety of acute "stressful" situations. However, steroids are not the major factor mediating eosinopenia associated with inflammation.

Eosinopenia is expected with most severe, ongoing inflammatory processes. It develops within hours of the onset of inflammation and disappears quickly as the inflammation subsides. Eosinopenia is so common with acute bacterial infections that such a diagnosis should be questioned if eosinophils are found easily on the blood smear. The cause of the initial eosinopenia is multifactorial, reflecting loss of blood eosinophils to the inflamed area, cessation of their release from marrow, and perhaps margination, as well as return from blood to marrow. Initially, the number of eosinophils in the bone marrow increases, but as inflammation persists, eosinophil production and eosinophils in marrow both decline. With most types of induced inflammations, migrating eosinophils remain in the periphery of the inflamed tissue and only a few accompany the neutrophils and monocytes into the exudate itself.

EOSINOPHIL FUNCTION. The overall pattern of marrow production, adhesion, migration, attachment, phagocytosis, and killing that was outlined for neutrophils is applicable to eosinophils. However, when the two are challenged in the same *in vitro* tests, either one or both may respond. When compared with the neutrophil, the eosinophil generally is sluggish and inefficient in phagocytosis and killing of bacteria. As noted above, eosinophils move into virtually any type of induced inflammation, often remaining in its periphery, and their function in most inflammations is unknown. Eosinophils will phagocytose and kill most bacteria but do not seem to have much overall importance in bacterial defense.

The eosinophil's role in *metazoan infections,* particularly in schistosomiasis, has been moderately well elucidated. In general, studies of other helminthic infections that are associated with eosinophilia indicate a similar role for eosinophils to that shown for schistosoma; they are essential for fighting larvae that are invading tissues, but are of little benefit or even detrimental to tissues with established parasites.

In schistosomiasis, extreme degrees of eosinophilia may be present (i.e., more than 100,000 eosinophils per mm^3), although lesser degrees are much more common. Neutrophilia often is also present, and while both types of cells and monocytes migrate into the infected tissue, eosinophils tend to predominate. Eosinophils are relatively ineffective against larvae unless the host has been immunized by previous infection. However, if the larvae have been coated by specific IgG (also IgE), or if complement is activated on its surface, the eosinophil becomes a fairly efficient aggressor. This presumably is mediated by eosinophil membrane receptor sites for the Fc portion of IgG and IgE and for complement, and these receptors as well as eosinophil migration are enhanced by products of mast cells.

The eosinophil does not actually phagocytose the larva, which is much larger than its attacker. However, it uses the same overall mechanism to attack and kill as it would presumably use could it ingest the larva. In the presence of Ig or activated complement on the larval surface, the eosinophil adheres to it and molds its adherent surface to an exact copy of the larval surface. Granules fuse with one another, then with the adherent eosinophil membrane, and thus, granule contents are released into the potential space between the eosinophil and the worm.

Eosinophil granules are quite different from those of neutrophils. By electron microscopy they contain a crystalloid structure, surrounded by an amorphous matrix, while the interior of neutrophil granules is fairly homogeneous in structure. In the neutrophil, granule synthesis ceases after the myelocyte stage, but even "mature" eosinophils that have migrated into nonmyeloid tissue can continue to synthesize small, dense, enzyme-rich granules. Peroxidase is a major granule matrix component, as in the primary granule of neutrophils, but it is a different peroxidase. The crystalloid contains small cationic proteins and a major basic pattern. Eosinophils lack lysozyme but contain significantly more peroxidase, β-glucuronidase, acid phosphatase, arylsulfatase, and phospholipases than do neutrophils.

Granule contents damage and degrade the larval wall, and as lesions are created, the eosinophil sends processes into the worm, releasing more granules. The basic and cationic proteins have larvocidal properties for schistosomes (and also for trichinella). Thus, eosinophils are effective in preventing, or at least reducing, the penetration of larvae in previously sensitized hosts.

However, their role in certain types of established infections may be detrimental rather than helpful to the host. The granulomatous reaction by which the eggs of schistosomes are surrounded is one of the principal causes of tissue damage in hepatic schistosomiasis. Eosinophils are an active part of these granulomas and, in fact, can kill at least a portion of the eggs. However, the eosinophil activity in the lesion must contribute to granuloma formation; eosinophil ablation with antisera not only reduces the size of egg-associated granulomas, but decreases the associated hepatocellular damage.

In general, eosinophils are more effective against trematodes and cestodes than nematodes. However, the damage done to the surface of worms that they themselves do not kill may aid the attack of neutrophils, monocytes, and macrophages.

Allergic reactions, particularly the immediate-type hypersensitivity reactions, are characterized by infiltration of the reacting tissues with eosinophils, and often are associated with eosinophilia. Immunologically challenged mast cells (see below), probably activated by specific IgE, lymphocytes, and perhaps other cells, release a variety of substances that are chemotactic for eosinophils and that otherwise "activate" the eosinophil. The eosinophil probably does not in any sense induce the allergic response, but rather functions to control it, in large part by modulating the effect of activated mast cells (Table 6). However, the same eosinophil constituents that neutralize or degrade reaction products of mast cells can also damage normal tissue. Thus, containment of the allergic response may be associated with other, and adverse, effects. The eosinophil is an efficient and somewhat selective phagocyte for antigen-antibody complexes that play an integral role in damage associated with certain of the allergic reactions. However, the utility, if any, of this eosinophil activity in such reactions is undefined.

Idiopathic forms of eosinophilia are poorly understood and have been referred to by many terms, perhaps most commonly simply as "hypereosinophilic syndromes," or "eosinophilic leukemia." Certain of these do appear to be clonal neoplastic diseases of the myeloid stem cell system, primarily expressed by increased production of eosinophils, and thus can be properly termed leukemia. In others, high serum levels of IgE suggest that the eosinophilia may be in response to an undefined immune reaction. Some patients with idiopathic, hypereosinophilic syndromes remain asymptomatic for many years, but others suffer from recurrent pulmonary infiltration and thrombophlebitis, and often die with intractable congestive heart failure. The heart failure is due to endocardial fibrosis, and this fibrosis may be due to the damaging effect of a released substance from eosinophils (? major basic protein). In patients with eosinophilia and endomyocardial fibrosis, more degranulated eosinophils are in the blood than in persons without such fibrosis. It seems unlikely that the eosinophilia is simply in reaction to an undefined pathogenic event in the endocardium, for such fibrosis has been seen not only with idiopathic disease but also with "tropical eosinophilia" (associated with filaria), eosinophilia associated with cancer of the lung, and with other diseases.

BASOPHILS AND MAST CELLS

The granules of neutrophils were termed "suicide bags" by Hirsch when he first described degranulation. This was based on the observation that release of the

TABLE 6. Certain Effects of Eosinophils upon Mast Cells and Mast Cell Products in the Immediate-Type Delayed Hypersensitivity Allergic Reaction

Inhibits release of mediators from mast cells, perhaps by influencing intracellular prosta-
glandin concentration.
Phagocytoses released mast cell granules.
Secretes:
Major basic protein (neutralizes heparin)
Histaminase
Lysophospholipase
Arylsulfatase B (degrades slow-reacting substance of anaphylaxis)
Phospholipase D (degrades platelet lytic factor).

cell's granule content into its cytoplasm was associated with cell death, although he later showed that intracytoplasmic granule rupture was a part of cell death rather than its cause. However, "suicide bags" would be an appropriate term for the granules of basophils and mast cells since they can quickly kill the host in which the cell resides. Massive release of granule contents from these cells produces *sudden death* (anaphylactic shock). Rattlesnakes, cottonmouth moccasins, coral snakes, and copperheads are greatly feared by many persons, but deaths from allergic reactions due to wasp stings are much more common in the United States than are deaths from snake bites.

The basophil differs somewhat in appearance from the mast cell; it is smaller and has a segmented rather than round nucleus. The two may have minor differences in chemical composition. In the past, it was "popular" to consider them to be similar but entirely unrelated cellular systems. However, in the past few years, it has become increasingly clear that they share a fairly well differentiated myeloid stem cell and behave in virtually identical fashion with respect to their function in immune and inflammatory responses. Thus, we will discuss them together. Numerically, mast cells vastly exceed basophils; there are as many or more mast cells in 100 g of skin or lung as there are basophils in the entire blood and marrow. Basophils are produced in marrow via the same general manner outlined for neutrophils, although little is known of their kinetics. Tissue mast cells are exceedingly long lived; in normal rodents, their life span may be at least half that of the animal. In the adult, under most circumstances, an increase in tissue mast cells reflects *in situ* replication of existing cells or of resident precursors, but under certain circumstances of sudden and significant demand, they are derived from circulating progenitors of marrow origin.

Mast cells are mediators of inflammatory processes, particularly those initiated by hypersensitivity reactions. In the presence of a variety of specific stimuli, mast cells release a witches' brew of enzymes, proteoglycans, and other substances that are vasoactive, bronchoconstrictive, and chemotactic (especially for eosinophils) (Table 7). In the allergic response, two molecules of IgE, bound to mast cell receptors, are bridged by the specific antigen. This initiates a series of membrane and intracellular events that culminate in fusion of granule and cytoplasmic membrane with release of granule contents, or in formation of a phagosome-like structure that contains and releases intact granules. The degranulated mast cell can then synthesize a new complement of granules. Many of the major mast cell dependent mediators attract or enhance the attraction of eosinophils and in turn are modified by eosinophils and eosinophil products (see page 56). As Austin noted, "The eosinophil can undo what the mast cell does."

Basophilia (finding them easily on a blood smear) usually is indicative of one of the clonal, myeloid stem cell tumors (see page 15). Modest degrees of basophilia may be seen with inflammatory bowel diseases and with myxedema. Increased tissue mast cells are present in idiopathic, congenital, and acquired forms, and in some instances mast cell infiltration is very prominent. In the last case, the term systemic mastocytosis has been applied. When mast cells are in blood, it has been termed mast cell leukemia.

TABLE 7. Certain Mast-Cell-Dependent Mediators

Mediator:	
Released as Preformed Substance	
Histamine	Smooth muscle contraction
	Increase in vascular permeability
	Modulation of chemotaxis, prostaglandins, cyclic nucleotides
Serotonin	Smooth muscle contraction
	Increase in vascular permeability
Eosinophil chemotactic factors (various)	Attract and deactivate eosinophils and neutrophils
Heparin	Anticoagulation
	Neutralizes major basic proteins of eosinophils
Enzymes (chymase, peroxidase, arylsulfatase, and so forth)	Proteolysis, hydrolysis, cleavage, and so forth
Chondroitin sulfate	Interacts with platelets
Newly Generated on Release	
Leukotrienes (slow-reacting substances of anaphylaxis)	Smooth muscle contraction
	Increase in vascular permeability
	Chemotactic
	Modulates histamine, prostaglandins
Platelet activating factor	Promotes platelet aggregation, adhesion, and so forth
Preformed and/or Generated	
Prostaglandins and other arachidonic metabolites	Smooth muscle contraction and relaxation
	Chemotaxis
	Modulate cyclic nucleotides

5

LYMPHOCYTES AND
THE IMMUNE SYSTEM

Lymphocytes, which constitute the second most numerous white cell in peripheral blood, are essential components of the immune defense system. Their primary function is to react with antigens and thus initiate immune responses. It is not surprising that diseases affecting lymphocytes frequently manifest themselves either as an inability to protect the individual against environmental pathogens (*immune deficiency disorders*) or as the development of immune reactions directed against antigens on the individual's own cells (*autoimmune diseases*). In this chapter, the characteristics of lymphocytes, as presently understood, are discussed. However, it is important to recognize that these concepts are areas of intense investigation. As new information accumulates, many of these concepts will require further modification and reinterpretation.

The blood-borne lymphocytes represent only a small fraction of the total body pool of these cells, probably less than 5 percent. The majority are located in the spleen, lymph nodes, and other organized lymphatic tissues. In contrast to neutrophils, most of the blood lymphocytes are able to enter and leave the circulation freely. As such, there is a continuous movement of cells from one area or compartment to another. This process is called *recirculation*. Despite this complex circulation, the entire system is normally maintained in equilibrium, and, in the steady state, the number of lymphocytes in the blood and tissues is kept quite constant.

Most lymphocytes in both the blood and the lymphatic tissues are recognized as small cells without unique morphologic features (see page 4). They may be viewed as intermitotic or resting cells that have been reduced to the smallest possible size to permit easy mobility. Larger lymphoid cells (medium and large lymphocytes) are usually present as a minor population. Most of these larger cells are believed to be derived from small lymphocytes and probably represent immunologically active cells that are responding to or have recently responded to antigenic challenges.

Despite their morphologic similarities, lymphocytes comprise several functionally distinct subpopulations. Based on their predominant immunologic activity, two major classes of lymphocytes have been defined—T (thymic dependent) lymphocytes, which are primarily responsible for *cell-mediated immune reactions,* and B (bone marrow derived) lymphocytes, which are capable of synthesizing immunoglobulins and are themselves precursors of plasma cells (*humoral immune reactions*). In addition, there is a third group of lymphocytes that lack characteristics of either T or B cells. These are collectively referred to as *null* cells. Recent studies indicate that these lymphocytes are a mixture of several different types of cells; certain subtypes appear to have important immunologic activities.

FUNCTIONAL DIVISION OF THE IMMUNE SYSTEM

As lymphocytes are primarily concerned with maintenance of the immune defense system, an appreciation of the general types of immunologic reactions is essential to an understanding of lymphoid physiology and pathology. There are two general types of responses, cell-mediated and humoral. The former requires direct cell contact between the antigen and the effector lymphocyte; the reaction occurs at the local site and generally develops slowly. Serum factors are not required. In most cases, T lymphocytes are the effector cells. However, specific forms of cell-mediated reactions that result in target-cell lysis can also be effected by null cells (see discussion later in this chapter).

Humoral reactions involve the synthesis and secretion of antibodies, which are specifically modified proteins capable of reacting selectively with the inciting antigen. As a group, antibodies are collectively referred to as *immunoglobulins.* Humoral reactions can occur at sites distal to the cells synthesizing the specific antibodies. Therefore, direct contact between antigen and the effector cells is not required. Effectors of humoral responses are B lymphocytes and their progeny, plasma cells. In many reactions, mediators of inflammation, such as complement components, are essential cofactors. It should be noted that most antigens evoke both a cell-mediated response and a humoral response. However, in a functioning immune defense system, each form of immunity is predominantly responsible for certain protective activities, and each can mediate distinct pathologic abnormalities. The major roles of each are summarized in Table 8.

A prime function of the immune defense system is that of providing protection against environmental pathogens. Each immune component is considered to have a dominant role in the resistance to certain classes of infectious agents. With respect to bacteria, humoral immunity is concerned principally with the resistance to encapsulated, pyogenic organisms (pneumococci, streptococci,

TABLE 8. Major Activities of Humoral and Cellular Immunity

Humoral Immunity
1. Elimination of encapsulated bacteria.
2. Neutralization of soluble toxins; viral protection (incubation phase).
3. Transplantation rejection (hyperacute reaction).
4. ? Tumor immunity.
5. Immunologically-related diseases (autoimmune blood dyscrasia, "toxic complex" diseases, allergic disorders).

Cellular Immunity
1. Resistance against intracellular pathogens (many bacteria, most viruses, protozoa, fungi).
2. Transplantation rejection (acute and chronic reactions).
3. Tumor immunity.
4. Autoimmunity (role not well defined).
5. Contact dermatitis.

meningococci, and *H. influenzae*). Antibody coating of these organisms greatly facilitates their phagocytosis and subsequent destruction. The immune reaction also initiates the sequence of complement fixation and activation; these components further enhance bacterial elimination. Individuals with a marked deficiency in serum immunoglobulins are extremely susceptible to recurrent infections by this spectrum of organisms. Serum antibodies also participate in the protection against certain viral infections, especially during their incubation period, and are important in neutralizing soluble toxins (i.e., tetanus toxin).

Until recently, the role of cell-mediated immunity in the host defense system was largely unknown. It is now recognized that it represents the major immunologic reaction against intracellular pathogens. Included in this group are many bacteria, such as *Mycoplasm tuberculosis* and *Salmonella,* and most viruses, fungi, and protozoa. Other aspects of the role of cellular immunity are discussed below.

DEVELOPMENT OF THE LYMPHOID SYSTEM

Through studies of animal models and human immune deficiency diseases, the ontogeny of the lymphoid system has been partially defined (Fig. 22). In parallel with other cellular systems, lymphocytes develop from stem cells (see page 4). At this stage of development, these stem cells are *immunologically incompetent* in that they lack the ability to initiate immune responses.

A proportion of lymphoid stem cells migrate from myeloid tissues to the thymus. In the thymus, they undergo both proliferative expansion and maturation into mature T cells. Thymopoiesis is an ineffective process; it appears that the vast majority of thymus lymphocytes die either within this organ itself or very shortly after emigrating from it. Only a small proportion seed the peripheral tissues as mature T cells, capable of effecting cell-mediated responses.

Two facets of thymic maturation are of importance. First, the thymus functions primarily during fetal life. In man, the peripheral T lymphoid system is fully developed at birth, and it does not require a constant input of new cells for

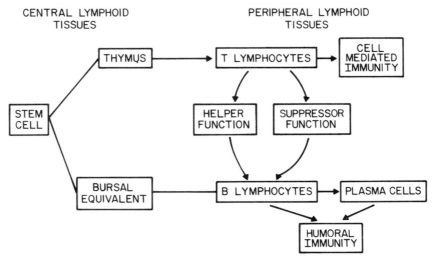

CENTRAL LYMPHOID TISSUES

PERIPHERAL LYMPHOID TISSUES

FIGURE 22. Development of the lymphoid system. The central lymphoid tissues contain immunologically immature cells; the peripheral tissues contain cells capable of effecting an immune response. No "bursa" has been identified in man and it is believed that maturation of B cells occurs in the myeloid tissues. Note that despite the apparent independent origins of both the T and B cells, these are highly interdependent systems (indicated by T help and T suppression of B cell responses).

maintenance during postnatal life. As such, it is possible to surgically remove the thymus without causing severe immunologic failure. Thymectomy is performed as treatment for diseases such as myasthenia gravis. Such individuals do not encounter severe impairment in their cell-mediated immune system. By contrast, failure of the thymus to develop during fetal life leads to a severe defect in cell-mediated immunity (*DiGeorge's syndrome*) usually resulting in death during infancy as a consequence of repeated infections.

Second, the maturation of stem cells to T lymphocytes in the thymus is believed to be governed by thymic humoral factors synthesized by epithelial elements of this organ. Several groups have isolated, characterized, and purified thymic hormones. These are now being utilized in clinical trials as possible therapeutic agents in diseases characterized by impaired cellular immunity.

The maturation of the B lymphoid system is less well defined. In birds, it is known that a hindgut lymphoid organ, the bursa of Fabricius, is responsible for the maturation of stem cells into B lymphocytes. No organ equivalent to the bursa has been identified in man, and, most likely, maturation of B cells occurs directly in the marrow and other hematopoietic tissues. (The term "B" lymphocyte arose from this bursal origin, but it is used currently in reference to maturation of B cells in the bone marrow.) The transformation of stem cells to mature B lymphocytes involves several intermediate stages; during these, the cells acquire the capabilities of synthesizing different types of immunoglobulins and express a series of cell membrane-associated receptors.

Although the classic models of immunity suggest that the T-cell and B-cell systems develop and function independently, the two are, in fact, very interdependent. This is best illustrated by considering T-cell control of humoral immunity. One subset of T cells (inducer or helper cells) is required to initiate many humoral responses. The T cells initially interact with the antigen and, in cooperation with macrophages, instruct B cells to respond. It is the B lymphocyte that ultimately develops into the antibody-synthesizing plasma cells. However, in response to most antigens, these B cells are unable to react in the absence of T-helper-cell influences. Most likely, this T-cell-helper activity is mediated by a soluble factor released by these lymphocytes. Antigens that require interactions between T cells and B cells for elaborating humoral responses are termed *thymic dependent;* a second and smaller number of antigens can directly stimulate B cells in the absence of T cells (*thymic independent antigens*).

A second level of interaction between T and B cells serves to regulate the magnitude of humoral responses. T-cell subsets distinct from the T helper cells (T suppressor cells) act to restrict the ability of B cells to produce antibodies to either thymic dependent or thymic independent antigens. This type of negative regulatory influence is of great importance both in terminating responses to foreign antigens and in maintaining *tolerance* (specific immunologic unresponsiveness) to self antigens. Tolerance prevents the immune defense system from mounting attacks against the individual's own antigens.

LYMPHOCYTE RESPONSES TO ANTIGEN

Mature lymphocytes undergo a coordinated series of morphological and biochemical changes when responding to specific antigen challenges (Fig. 23). Prior to contact with the stimuli, these cells exist as small, intermitotic lymphocytes. The interaction between antigens and responsive cells depends upon cell membrane-associated receptors; in the B cell system, these are membrane-bound immunoglobulins that have specificity for the antigen. Receptors on T cells have not been defined, but probably are similar to surface immunoglobulin receptors on B cells. These lymphocytes are now stimulated to become actively proliferating cells, thus, in a sense, again becoming stem cells. The cell enlarges, synthesizes new nucleic acids and proteins, and undergoes a series of mitoses. This proliferative expansion increases the pool of antigen-responsive cells. Following completion of this phase, daughter cells mature into immunologic effectors.

In the T cell system, these daughter cells are small lymphocytes that can mediate various effector functions. Additionally, some T cells act as memory cells; these are preprogrammed lymphocytes which, upon rechallenge with the inciting antigen, elicit a secondary or anamnestic-type immune response. Concomitantly, T cells elaborate a group of chemical mediators called "lymphokines," which serve to influence the activities of other cells. A representative, but incomplete, list of lymphokines is shown in Table 9. One of the most important targets of these lymphokines is macrophages. Soluble products of lymphocytes promote the attraction of macrophages to the site of antigen depo-

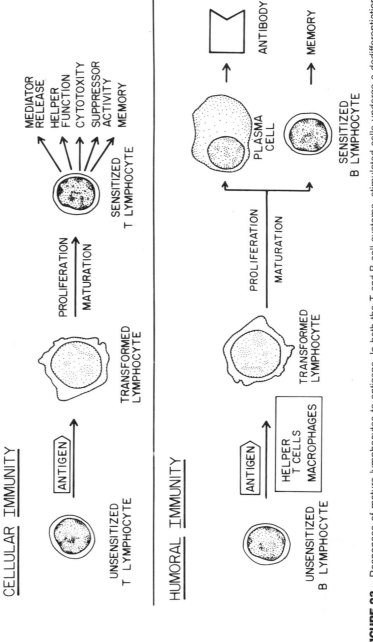

CELLULAR IMMUNITY

UNSENSITIZED
T LYMPHOCYTE

ANTIGEN

TRANSFORMED
LYMPHOCYTE

PROLIFERATION

MATURATION

SENSITIZED
T LYMPHOCYTE

MEDIATOR
RELEASE
HELPER
FUNCTION
CYTOTOXITY
SUPPRESSOR
ACTIVITY
MEMORY

HUMORAL IMMUNITY

UNSENSITIZED
B LYMPHOCYTE

ANTIGEN

HELPER
T CELLS
MACROPHAGES

TRANSFORMED
LYMPHOCYTE

PROLIFERATION

MATURATION

PLASMA
CELL

ANTIBODY

SENSITIZED
B LYMPHOCYTE

MEMORY

FIGURE 23. Responses of mature lymphocytes to antigens. In both the T and B cell systems, stimulated cells undergo a dedifferentiation process leading to immature-appearing lymphoblasts.

TABLE 9. Representative Lymphokine Activities

CELLULAR FUNCTION	MEDIATOR	ACTIVITY
Mobility	1. Chemotaxis—macrophages neutrophils, eosinophils, and basophils.	1. Attraction of cells to site of antigen deposition.
	2. Migration inhibition—macrophages (MIF), neutrophils (LIF).	2. Localizing inflammatory cells.
Injury	1. Lymphotoxin.	1. Killing of target cells.
Activation	1. Helper and suppressor factors.	1. Regulate activities of T and B cells.
	2. Macrophage activation factor (MAF).	2. Activate intracellular enzymes in macrophages.
	3. Augmentation of T-cell cytotoxicity.	3. Promotes target cell killing by T cells.
	4. Interferon.	4. Antiviral agent: increases NK activity.
	5. Stimulate collagen synthesis by fibroblasts.	5. Induces secretion of this extracellular matrix protein.
Growth	1. Mitogenic factor.	1. T-cell proliferation.
	2. T-cell growth factor (IL-2).	2. Perpetuates T-cell growth.
	3. Colony-stimulating factor (CSF).	3. Induces growth of neutrophils and macrophages.

sition (chemotactic factor), localize these phagocytic cells (migration-inhibiting factor, MIF), and enhance their ability to kill intracellular organisms (macrophage-activating factor). Simultaneously, the macrophages release their intracellular (lysosomal) enzymes; these cause the local inflammatory responses such as the erythema and induration seen in a delayed hypersensitivity skin test (see discussion later in this chapter). It should be noted that lymphokines generally are defined by biologic assays. Thus, it is not known whether all assays define separate and distinct lymphokines or whether some of these mediators have more than one activity.

On the basis of responses of T lymphocytes in culture, it appears that a complex interaction of soluble factors is involved in cell proliferation. One factor, *interleukin 1 (IL-1)*, is elaborated by monocytes; this soluble mediator may be of importance in the initial transformation of T cells into actively proliferating cells. The second factor, *interleukin 2 (IL-2)*, is produced by T cells and appears to be important in perpetuating the continued growth of previously-stimulated T lymphocytes. *In vitro*, IL-2 permits the long-term culture of these cells; as such, this factor has also been termed *T-cell growth factor*. From these observations, one model of T-cell growth *in vivo* can be depicted as follows. Antigen initially interacts with monocytes, inducing the release of IL-1. This factor, along with the antigen, then interacts with responsive T lymphocytes. One T-cell subset is activated to respond to the inciting antigen; a second subset is stimulated to release IL-2, which serves to promote the proliferative expansion of the effector population. In addition to T-cell proliferation, both IL-1 and IL-2 have other biologic activities; these include ability to mediate T-B cell interactions and to effect a broad range of lymphoid and nonlymphoid cell functions. This scheme is now being employed to generate clones of human T cells. In the future, it may be possible to use these clones therapeutically.

The initial stages of B-lymphocyte responses to antigens are quite similar (see Fig. 23). As noted above, in most reactions, stimulation requires the coordinated efforts of T helper cells and macrophages to initiate a B-cell response. Once appropriately stimulated, the B cell undergoes activation changes similar to those described for T lymphocytes. These include dedifferentiation, proliferation, and subsequent maturation. However, in the B cell system, the final effectors are plasma cells specifically modified for optimal secretion of antibodies with specificity for the inciting antigen. In addition, some of the daughter cells revert to small B lymphocytes; these serve as memory cells (stem cells for potential, future antigenic challenges).

T Lymphocytes

As noted above, these cells are responsible primarily for protection against intracellular pathogens; individuals who are grossly deficient in T-cell immunity frequently succumb to overwhelming infections by organisms such as cytomegalovirus, *Pneumocystis carinii*, *Candida*, and other apparently "opportunistic" bacteria, viruses and fungi. T-cell immunity is also the major mechanism for rejection of allogeneic tissue or organ transplants—in fact, the major limitation to transplant therapy has been the difficulty in suppressing T-cell allograft rejection reactions without overly compromising vital protective mechanisms. A form of immune reaction seen after bone marrow transplantation, graft-versus-host disease (GVHD), is also mediated by T lymphocytes. GVHD occurs when the transplant recipient is unable to reject an allograft of immunologically competent T cells. However, the grafted lymphocytes are capable of recognizing host antigens as foreign and developing immune responses against these antigens. Clinically, GVHD has been a major limitation to bone marrow transplantation; in its severest form, it is fatal.

There has been much discussion concerning the role of T cells in the immunologic protection against cancer. At one time, it was widely held that T-lymphocyte immunity was a prime protection mechanism. Acording to this thesis, tumor specific antigens (TSA) are capable of eliciting a response by cytotoxic T cells, which, in turn, destroy the tumor cells. Although it is likely that T-cell anti-tumor mechanisms exist both in animals and man, several recent studies have cast doubt as to their importance. Other immunologically-related cell-mediated cytolytic mechanisms, such as those expressed by NK or K cells (see discussion later in this chapter), appear to be of greater importance.

As described previously, T cells have an important role in humoral antibody production. One subset of these cells acts as helper/inducer lymphocytes that instruct B cells to respond to thymic-dependent antigens. Other T cells serve a suppressor function in limiting the magnitude of the response. T-suppressor-cell function also serves to modulate many responses by other populations of T cells.

T cells also have been implicated in the genesis of many autoimmune diseases. However, their precise role in the pathogenesis of these diseases is unknown. It has been established that these cells mediate reactions such as contact sensitivity (e.g., poison ivy rash). In addition, investigators have found an abundance of T cells in the affected tissues in many autoreactive pathologic states. However, the contribution of these cells to the initiation or perpetuation of the abnormal processes is, at present, unclear.

DELAYED HYPERSENSITIVITY TESTING. In man, the most common means of assessing T-cell activity *in vivo* is reactivity in delayed hypersensitivity skin tests. These reactions involve responses to antigens to which the individual previously has acquired sensitization. Upon intradermal injection of minute amounts of the specific antigen, a delayed-type cutaneous response occurs; this consists of erythema and induration at the site of injection. Typically, the lesion appears 24 to 48 hours after challenge. Histologically, it is characterized by an infiltration of lymphocytes and macrophages. The reaction to tuberculin protein in sensitized individuals is the prototype of a delayed hypersensitivity reaction. However, as the incidence of this infection declines, most normal individuals are not sensitized to these antigens and thus cannot react. Clinical testing of delayed hypersensitivity now employs several common antigens that elicit positive delayed hypersensitivity tests in most normal individuals. These antigens include *Candida,* mumps, and streptokinase-streptodornase. An inability to respond to any one of a battery of delayed hypersensitivity skin tests is termed *anergy;* this abnormality reflects either a temporary or permanent failure of cell-mediated immunity.

T CELL IDENTIFICATION. *In vitro,* T lymphocytes are generally recognized by their ability to form rosettes with sheep erythrocytes (E^+). In this assay, sheep red cells adhere selectively to the cell membrane of T lymphocytes; by contrast, they will not react to either B cells or null lymphocytes. An alternate method for enumerating T cells is by measuring reactivity with a pan-T-cell monoclonal antibody (discussed below). With either technique, T cells are found to be the predominant lymphocyte in the peripheral blood; 60 to 80 percent of the circulating cells are T lymphocytes. Thus, lymphopenia usually indicates a decrease in the number of circulating T cells.

The circulating pool of T cells represents several functionally distinct categories of lymphocytes. One group, termed the inducer/helper subset, is responsible primarily for activating or amplifying the functions of other cells. The prime example of this activity is the triggering of B cells to produce specific antibodies in response to thymic-dependent antigens. In addition, T inducer cells also act to activate macrophages, thereby increasing their bactericidal and cytotoxic functions. In turn, these activated macrophages serve as the prime effectors in the killing reactions involving intracellular pathogens. More recently, it has been found that T inducer cells play an essential role in amplifying the functions of other T cells and also have influences over a wide variety of nonlymphoid cells. The multiple activities of T inducer cells are depicted in Figure 24.

The second subset of T cells comprises two types of effectors, T suppressor cells and T cytotoxic cells. As noted above, T suppressor cells regulate the magnitude of immune responses. Sensitized T cytotoxic cells are capable of directly killing targets such as tumor cells or those infected with viruses. At present, it is not known whether the T suppressor cells and T cytotoxic cells are two different cell populations identified by the same antigen marker or one population of effectors with multiple potentials.

Two newly-developed assays have enabled the morphologic recognition of T-cell subsets. The first depends upon the presence of different immunoglobulin receptors on T-helper and T-suppressor subsets. T helper cells bear receptors for IgM, T suppressor cells for IgG. These two populations have been designated Tμ and Tγ, respectively. Recent studies, however, indicate that these techniques may not provide clear distinctions between subsets; receptors may change in culture systems; suppression in some assays has been reported to be mediated by IgM-bearing T cells, and many of the Tγ cells may be of monocyte origin.

MONOCLONAL ANTIBODIES. The second technique for phenotypically identifying T-cell subsets utilizes the newly-developed procedure for generating monoclonal antibodies. Monoclonal antibodies constitute a single species of immunoglobulins with specificity for a single antigen. They are produced by hybridization of mouse myeloma cells with antibody-producing murine spleen cells. The latter are elicited by immunizing mice with specific antigens. The myeloma cells impart to the hybrid the property of continuous growth, and the

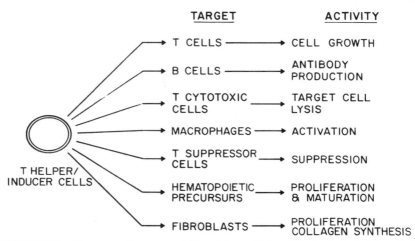

FIGURE 24. Diagrammatic representation of the multiple cell types that are influenced by products of stimulated T helper/inducer cells.

antibody-producing cells impart the ability to elaborate a single specific antibody. Once formed, the hybrid cell is cloned in order to generate large numbers of daughter cells, each with the same immunologic capacity. By selection, it is possible to obtain clones of hybrids that grow continuously and produce monoclonal antibodies to specific determinants of the immunizing antigens. Many monoclonal antibodies to T-cell subsets have now been developed and are now providing important clinical information as to the numbers and functions of these cells.

The most commonly-employed monoclonal antibodies to T-cell subsets are designated T3, T4, and T8. The T3 is a pan-T-cell reagent that can react with a determinant present on all peripheral T lymphocytes. T4 antibodies identify the T-inducer/helper subsets; the T8 antisera react with the cytotoxic/suppressor cell populations. In normal individuals, approximately 65 percent of circulating T cells are T4; the remaining 35 percent are T8. Thus, the ratio of T4 to T8 is approximately 2 to 1. Of note, altered ratios of T4 to T8 have been reported in many pathologic states. In general, several congenital and acquired immune deficiency diseases are characterized by a reduced ratio, whereas there is often an increased ratio in autoimmune diseases. Such observations suggest that normal immune reactivity is regulated by a balance between these two T-cell subsets (Fig. 25). Either an immune deficiency syndrome or an autoimmune syndrome could result from an alteration in the ratio of helper to suppressor cells. For example, an inability to respond to environmental antigens could result from either a deficiency in helper cell activity or an excess amount of suppres-

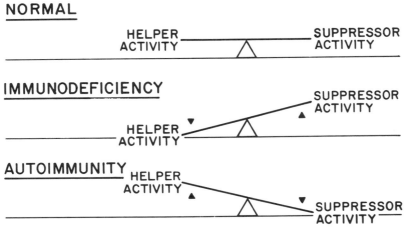

FIGURE 25. In normal individuals, there is a balance between helper and suppressor activities. Many immunodeficiency syndromes appear to result from a disturbance of this balance such that a state of unresponsiveness is created. This could result from either a lack of helper activity (↓ T4 cells) or an excess of suppressor activities (↑ T8 cells). Conversely, autoimmunity, which results from aberrant responses directed at host's own antigens, could result from abnormal immunoregulation from either excessive helper or reduced suppressor activities.

sion. Phenotypically, this would be typified by a decrease in T4 cells or an increase in T8 cells. Similarly, autoimmune diseases could develop from an excessive number of T4 helper cells or a lack of normally-occurring T8 suppressor cells. Examples of disorders in which imbalances between T inducer cells and T suppressor cells occur are shown in Table 10.

Monoclonal antibodies have been useful in tracing cell maturation through the thymus and providing important correlations between normal maturation and T-cell leukemias and lymphomas. Several different antigens appear sequentially and disappear as lymphocytes mature within the thymus. This is depicted in Figure 26. The earliest-appearing cell in the thymus contains the T10 antigen, a determinant also found on bone marrow cells. Some of the lymphoid cells in the thymus simultaneously manifest a second, early differentiation antigen, T9. Cells bearing either the T10 antigen alone or the T9 and T10 antigens in combination comprise about 10 percent of the thymic cellularity and are considered to be the most immature thymocytes. Approximately 80 percent of the cases of acute T-cell lymphoblastic leukemia bear only the T10 or the T9 and T10 antigens, suggesting that the neoplastic cells arise from these early thymocytes.

The majority of thymocytes show the following antigen composition: T10, T6, T4, and T8. Of these, the T6 antigen is a common thymus antigen; the T4 and T8 antigens denote the inducer (helper) and suppressor functions, respectively. It is noteworthy that at this stage of maturation, T cells appear to be programmed to differentiate along either functional pathway. These thymocytes comprise approximately 80 percent of the cells in the thymus, and at this stage of maturation, they lack immunologic reactivity. Anatomically, these cells are localized primarily in the cortical region of the thymus. Twenty percent of T-cell

TABLE 10.   Disorders Associated with Abnormal T-Cell Subsets

Immune Deficiency Diseases (Helper and/or Suppressor Activity)
 1. Common variable hypogammaglobulinemia.
 2. Acute viral infections (infectious mononucleosis, cytomegalic inclusion disease).
 3. Chronic graft-versus-host disease.
 4. Multiple myeloma.
 5. Chronic lymphocytic leukemia.
 6. Primary biliary cirrhosis.
 7. Sarcoidosis.
 8. Immunosuppressive drugs (azathioprine, corticosteroids, cyclosporin A.)

Autoimmunity (Helper and/or Suppressor Activity)
 1. Connective tissue diseases (systemic lupus erythematosus).
 2. Acute graft-versus-host disease.
 3. Autoimmune hemolytic anemia.
 4. Multiple sclerosis.
 5. Myasthenia gravis.
 6. Inflammatory bowel diseases.
 7. Atopic eczema.

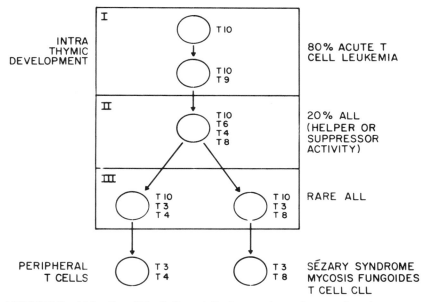

FIGURE 26. Maturation of T cells through the thymus. As can be seen, there is progressive acquisition and loss of antigens in association with cellular development. Different types of T-cell neoplasms can be equated with arrest at various stages of maturation.

acute lymphoblastic leukemia (ALL) and most cases of T-cell lymphoblastic lymphoma have phenotypes similar to these thymocytes.

During the last recognizable stages of intrathymic maturation, the T6 antigen is lost and the T3 antigen, characteristic of mature T cells, is acquired. During this phase of development, T cells differentiate into separate populations, one bearing only the T4 antigen and the other bearing the T8 antigen. However, they still differ from peripheral T lymphocytes in that they continue to express the T10 antigen. These mature thymocytes have acquired immunologic competence; anatomically, they are localized primarily in the medullary region of the thymus. Cases of T-cell CLL, lymphoblastic leukemia, and, rarely, cells from patients with Sezary syndrome and mycosis fungoides (the cutaneous T-cell lymphomas) bear this phenotype.

It should be recognized that thymocyte production is an example of highly ineffective lymphopoiesis. A relatively large number of precursors enter the thymus, and within the thymus, they have a very high rate of cell proliferation. Nevertheless, only a few cells ultimately develop into mature T cells populating peripheral tissues. This suggests that most die either within the thymus or shortly after migrating from this organ; less than 1 percent of thymocytes may actually develop into mature T cells.

B Lymphocytes

Humoral immunity, the expression of the functional activity of B lymphocytes, has as its major physiologic function the role of protection against encapsulated bacteria. Pathologically, aberrant antibody production is responsible for several immunologically-related diseases. These include immune destruction of blood cells (e.g., autoimmune hemolytic anemia, immune thrombocytopenia and neutropenia, and transfusion reactions), neutralization of serum proteins, toxic complex diseases (soluble antigen-antibody complexes such as those responsible for several forms of glomerulonephritis and vasculitis), and allergic diseases.

The role of immunoglobulins in transplant rejection reactions and tumor immunity has not been delineated fully. In transplants, antibodies are responsible for the hyperacute rejection reaction, the destruction of an organ occurring immediately after vascularization. Tumors may also be destroyed by antibodies, perhaps by an antibody-dependent cellular cytotoxicity (ADCC) mechanism (see discussion later in this chapter). By contrast, humoral antibodies can serve paradoxically to protect both transplanted organs and tumors by blocking destructive cell-mediated responses; this phenomenon is termed *immunologic enhancement.*

B CELL IDENTIFICATION. Recognition of B lymphocytes depends upon the property of these cells to synthesize immunoglobulins. Only small amounts are produced; these are incorporated into the cell membrane where they act as receptors for antigens. Identification is accomplished by reacting lymphocyte suspensions with heterologous antisera to immunoglobulins that have been labeled with a dye such as fluorescein. The antisera specifically combine with B cells, and when the suspension is examined by fluorescent microscopy, only B lymphocytes appear as reactive cells. Using this technique, it appears that B cells comprise 5 to 10 percent of the circulating pool of lymphocytes. Most B lymphocytes bear surface IgM antibodies; some simultaneously express both IgM and IgD. A small percent of B lymphocytes are positive for either IgG or IgA. Regardless of the types of immunoglobulins expressed by a lymphocyte, it appears that each B cell is monoclonal in that it will react with only a single antigenic determinant.

B CELL DEVELOPMENT. Recent studies have defined several stages in the ontogeny of B lymphocytes (Fig. 27). These cells arise from specific precursors, pre-B cells, which develop in hematopoietic tissues. Pre-B cells are found in the human fetal liver during the eighth week of gestation; during the 12th week, they are also found in the bone marrow. Recognizable B cells are identified in each organ approximately one to two weeks after the appearance of pre-B cells. During fetal life, pre-B cells are quite numerous; they are present in quantities equal to the number of B cells. After birth, however, they continue to be present but in smaller numbers. Pre-B cells comprise about 1 percent of the nucleated bone marrow cells in adults.

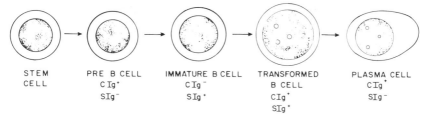

| STEM CELL | PRE B CELL cIg^+ sIg^- | IMMATURE B CELL cIg^- sIg^+ | TRANSFORMED B CELL cIg^+ sIg^+ | PLASMA CELL cIg^+ sIg^- |

FIGURE 27. B-cell maturation from stem cells. The "pre-B cell" is identified by the intracytoplasmic presence of the μ heavy chain of immunoglobulins (cIg^+). As the cell matures, it expresses immunoglobulins on its cell surface (sIg^+) but loses the detectable cytoplasmic component. The end-stage plasma cell has intracellular Ig (cIg^+) but lacks surface Ig (sIg^-).

Pre-B cells have unique characteristics. They show small quantities of cytoplasmic immunoglobulins (cIg), which are identified as portions of the IgM molecule ($cIgM$). At this stage, they lack cell-surface-associated immunoglobulins (sIg). As such, these cells are designated $cIgM^+ sIg^-$. Recent studies suggest that these cells may bear only μ heavy chains; an associated light chain appears to be absent. Of note, it appears that, at this early stage, the cell is committed to react with a single specific antigen. This suggests that antigen reactivity is determined very early in the cell's ontogeny.

Morphologically, the early pre-B cell is identified as a large lymphoid cell that is replicating rapidly. As the cell matures, it assumes the appearance of a small lymphocyte which is still $cIgM^+ sIg^-$. The next stage of development, which may occur while the cell is in the marrow or after it has migrated to the peripheral tissues, involves a loss of recognizable cytoplasmic immunoglobulins and the appearance of surface IgM (sIg^+). Development of the cell to this stage occurs entirely independently of exogenous antigenic stimulation.

Further maturation is a complex process in which the cells simultaneously express IgM and IgD. Some cells mature further into lymphocytes bearing either IgG or IgA. During this process, B cells also develop other membrane determinants. These include receptors for the Fc proportion of IgG, complement receptors (C3b and C3d), products of a major histocompatibility complex (Ia-like antigens), and receptors for T-cell-activating factors.

The final stages of maturation result in the conversion of B cells to plasma cells. The latter are specifically modified cells capable of synthesizing and secreting large quantities of specific antibodies. During this process, reacting lymphocytes lose their surface immunoglobulins but contain large quantities of cytoplasmic antibodies. Cellular counterparts of virtually all stages of B-cell maturation are identified in the different forms of lymphocytic neoplasms (see page 89).

Null Cells

Lymphocytes lacking surface immunoglobulins (sIg^-) and receptors for sheep red blood cells (E^-) have been designated collectively as *null cells*. These are a heterogeneous group of lymphocytes that include both precursor cells and those with specific immunologic activities. The immune functions include two recently recognized forms of cell-mediated cytolysis, natural killing and antibody-dependent cellular cytotoxicity.

Natural killer cells, which have been identified tentatively in man as "large granular lymphocytes," comprise a group of lymphoid cells that spontaneously kill tumor or viral infected cells. The activity of these cells differs from T-cell-mediated cytotoxicity by several criteria. One of the most important is the cellular requirement for prior sensitization. T cells must be educated to effect cell-mediated lysis, whereas natural killer (NK) cells are able to act without initial sensitization. Furthermore, NK cells arise in the absence of the thymus, whereas T-cell cytotoxic effectors require this influence for development. Several studies suggest that there is a high correlation between levels of NK activity *in vitro* and resistance to specific tumor challenges *in vivo*. However, direct proof that these cells constitute an important resistance mechanism is not yet available.

Effectors of NK activity have not been characterized completely. By morphologic criteria, these cells are lymphocytes. Some effector cells may be pre-T cells; this is suggested by the presence of receptors for sheep red blood cells. However, NK effectors also react with a monoclonal antibody specific for monocytes (OKM1).

A second type of cytolytic effector is referred to as K or killer cells. These lymphoid-appearing cells have the ability to kill IgG-coated target cells directly; this reaction occurs in the absence of complement (Fig. 28). Like NK cells, K cells do not require prior antigenic exposure in order to effect target-cell killing. The cellular requirement for effecting this cytotoxic reaction is the presence of receptors for IgG on the effectors; these permit the binding of the K cells to the target cell. Once direct cell contact has been established, the effector lymphocyte is then capable of delivering a lytic injury. The killing reaction has been termed antibody-dependent cellular cytotoxicity (ADCC). In addition to null lymphocytes, monocytes are also able to effect ADCC reactions.

There has been extensive speculation as to possible physiologic roles for K cells. However, their function to date has not been defined fully. It has been postulated that they serve an important role in eliminating tumors and virally infected cells. It has also been suggested that ADCC reactions may be responsible for several autoimmune disorders; in these processes, the effectors react

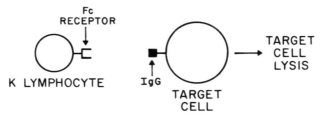

FIGURE 28. Antibody-dependent cellular cytotoxicity (ADCC). A type of null lymphocyte, termed the K cell, attaches to an IgG-coated target cell via Fc receptors on the K cell. This binding serves to permit the lymphocyte to effect a lytic attack on the target cell.

with antibody-coated "self" cells (e.g., thyroid cells coated with antithyroglobulin antibodies). Whether K cells and NK cells are separate populations or represent two activities effected by the same cell population is, at present, undefined.

LYMPHOCYTE RESPONSES IN CULTURE

Many of the functional activities of mature lymphocytes can be simulated *in vitro;* these assays have been of great value in the clinical assessment of immune function and in increasing our understanding of the pathophysiology of lymphoid diseases. A complete discussion of all *in vitro* tests is beyond the scope of this book. In essence, these cells can be studied for many functional properties, including their ability to elaborate mediators, act as suppressor cells, effect cytolytic reactions, and elaborate soluble helper factors.

One type of response that deserves particular mention is the ability of immunologically competent lymphocytes to proliferate *in vitro.* This type of reaction depends upon the presence of an exogenous stimulus, a mitogen. The most widely-used agents are designated as nonspecific mitogens because they are capable of inducing large numbers of cells to transform into actively proliferating lymphocytes. The response is independent of prior antigen sensitization. Examples of these agents are phytohemagglutinin (PHA), Concanavalin A (Con-A) and pokeweed mitogen. Of note, each mitogen appears to react with a distinct population of lymphocytes. PHA and Con-A are considered primarily stimuli for T-cell proliferation, although both can also react with B cells. Con-A has been shown to be particularly active in stimulating suppressor T cells. Pokeweed is a T-dependent B-cell mitogen; it activates both populations but has greater specificity for the latter. In addition to inducing proliferation, pokeweed can act to stimulate immunoglobulin synthesis nonspecifically by cultured B lymphocytes.

In addition to nonspecific mitogens, histoincompatible lymphocytes can also induce proliferative responses. Cells from two unrelated individuals will serve to stimulate each other; this test, the mixed lymphocyte culture (MLC), is used widely to type donors and recipients in preparation for organ transplantation. Lymphocytes from an individual sensitized to a specific antigen (e.g., tuberculin protein) are capable of responding to the antigen by proliferation. However, only a small fraction of cultured cells respond. Reactivity to these specific stimuli requires both presensitization of the cells and an intact effector mechanism.

LYMPHOCYTE LIFE SPAN

The heterogeneity of lymphocytes is manifest not only by differences in functional potential but also in terms of life span and turnover rates. By these kinetic criteria, lymphoid cells are classified as either long-lived or short-lived. Unfortunately, this division does not closely parallel the separation of cells into immunologic classes. There are both short- and long-lived T and B cells, a point which generally serves as a source of confusion.

Although both kinetic populations are present in the peripheral blood, the predominant cell type is a long-lived element. In most animal species, more than 80 percent of blood lymphocytes belong to this group; further, the vast majority of these long-lived cells are identified functionally as T cells. Several criteria distinguish these cells: they have a unique circulatory pattern such that they can both leave and reenter the circulation (*recirculation*); their transit time in the blood is rapid; and in both the blood and peripheral tissues, they can persist in a prolonged intermitotic or G_0 phase.

The life span of human lymphocytes has been calculated by assessing the disappearance rate of irradiation-induced chromosome abnormalities. Sublethal doses of irradiation cause specific chromosome injuries that are not deleterious to the cell as long as it persists in an intermitotic phase. However, these abnormalities are lethal when the cell divides. By serially measuring the disappearance rate of aberrations, it has been estimated that the average intermitotic interval is between two to four years, and a sizeable number of cells may survive without dividing for 10 years or longer.

Long-lived lymphocytes persist in the blood for only a brief period and then migrate directly through the cytoplasm of postcapillary or high endothelial venule cells and through cells lining the venules distal to these segments. In addition, migration can also occur directly through cells lining lymphatic channels. The lymphocytes tend to populate specific regions of lymphoid tissues (Fig. 29). T cells tend to localize in the paracortical regions of lymph nodes, the periarteriolar regions of the spleen, and the interfollicular regions of gut-associated lymphoid tissues. These areas have been termed *thymic-dependent zones*. By contrast, B cells migrate to the follicular and medullary regions of lymph nodes, the primary follicles and red pulp of the spleen, and the follicular regions of gut-associated lymphoid tissues (*thymic-independent regions*). Once localized, both types of recirculating cells persist as small intermitotic lymphocytes for an indeterminate time, but retain the capacity to re-enter the circulation. In the lymph nodes, this is accomplished by migration into the efferent lymphatic and then into the thoracic duct and other lymphatic-vascular connections. Lymphoid recirculation continues until the cell is stimulated by an appropriate antigen. This recirculation process is important in disseminating immunologic information throughout the body.

The major stimulus for both T- and B-cell replication is contact with environmental antigens. If exposure to antigens is minimized, as in animals reared from birth in a germ-free environment, the peripheral lymphatic system remains rudimentary. However, when these animals are exposed to a normal antigenic load, a rapid growth of the entire lymphoid system occurs.

LYMPHOCYTE ENZYMES

In addition to immunologic markers, biochemical characteristics of lymphocyte subsets have provided valuable information as to the origins, functions, and diversity of these cells. Several enzymes have clinical relevance. Of these, the most notable is the nuclear enzyme terminal deoxynucleotidyl transferase (TdT).

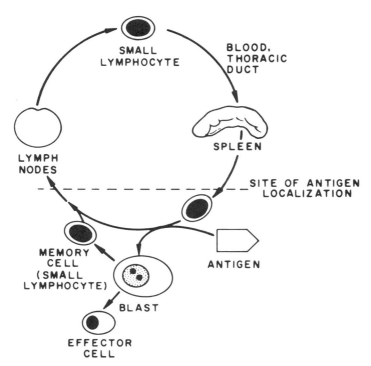

FIGURE 29. Lymphocyte recirculation. Mature cells migrate from between lymphoid tissues via the blood, hence these lymphocyte are capable of both entering and leaving the circulation. This process continues until the lymphocyte encounters an appropriate antigen, which induces it to transform and respond immunologically. Recirculation is an important activity as it serves to disseminate immunologic information throughout the body.

This is present in thymocytes, but is virtually undetectable in peripheral T or B lymphocytes. Of note, high concentrations are observed in many forms of acute lymphoblastic leukemia, and, recently, TdT has been found in the leukemic cells of approximately one third of individuals with the blasts crisis of CML (see page 19). This suggests a lymphocytic origin of these cells; the blast appears to arise from an early precursor common to both lymphocytic and hematopoietic systems.

Two forms of immune deficiency syndromes have been linked to enzyme deficiencies. Some patients with severe combined immunodeficiency lack the enzyme adenosine deaminase (ADA); this results in a failure of lymphocytes to synthesize purines and results in intracellular accumulation of the toxic metabolite deoxyadenosine. Affected patients suffer from severe defects in both the T- and B-cell systems.

A deficiency of another enzyme, purine nucleoside phosphorylase (PNP), also results in an immune deficiency, primarily affecting T cells. PNP is also involved in the metabolism of purines, and in affected patients, toxic concentrations of deoxyguanosine occur intracellularly.

Phosphatases are found in lymphocytes; in one disease, hairy-cell leukemia or leukemic reticuloendotheliosis, a distinct isoenzyme is present. This acid phosphatase is resistant to tartrate treatment. By contrast, the acid phosphatases in other lymphoproliferative diseases are sensitive to this manipulation.

The liposomal enzyme α-naphthyl acid esterase (ANAE) has proven to be a reliable marker for human T cells.

IMMUNOGLOBULINS

Immunoglobulins, a term used collectively to describe serum antibodies, are a heterogeneous group of proteins, each specifically modified to react with a particular antigen. Antibodies are synthesized primarily by plasma cells; however, small amounts are also produced by B lymphocytes. All antibodies of the same type that are specific for a single antigen are believed to be derived from a single clone of cells. A *clone* represents a population of cells all originating from a single common precursor; thus, each cell in a clone is programmed to respond by elaborating the same antibody.

Immunoglobulins (Ig) are subdivided into five classes, in order of decreasing concentrations: IgG, IgA, IgM, IgD, and IgE. (Properties of each class are shown in Table 11). Most antibodies belong to the IgG class. Further separation of IgG proteins indicates that four distinct subclasses are present; these are designated IgG_1, IgG_2, IgG_3, and IgG_4. Each subclass has slightly different bio-

TABLE 11. Properties of Immunoglobulins

	IgG	IgA	IgM	IgD	IgE
Serum concentration (mg/ml)	12.4	2.5	1.2	0.03	0.0003
Molecular weight	160,000	170,000 385,000*	900,000	180,000	200,000
Sedimentation coefficient	7S	7S (9S, 11S, 13S)	19S	7S	8S
Biological half life (days)	23†	6	5	2.8	2.4
Synthetic rate mg/kg/ day	34	24	3.3	0.4	0.0023
Percent intravascular	45	42	80	75	51
Biological function	principal serum antibody	secretory antibody	initial response to antigen	unknown	anaphylactic reaction

*The molecular weight of serum IgA is 170,000. Secretory IgA consists of two units of IgA combined with "secretory piece" (MW 385,000).

†Biological half life of IgG is a function of serum concentration; T½ is prolonged with low levels, shortened with high concentrations. Half lives of other immunoglobulins are independent of serum concentrations.

logic properties. For example, IgG₁ and IgG₃ are effective in activating complement via the classic pathway. However, IgG₂ is only minimally active in this reaction, and IgG₄ is unable to activate complement via the classic pathway. Both IgA and IgM can also be divided into several subclasses.

Although IgA is the immunoglobulin in the second highest concentration in the serum, its major physiologic role is in external secretions. This immunoglobulin predominates in lacrimal, nasopharyngeal, salivary, respiratory, and gastrointestinal fluids. Plasma cells located in the submucosa of these organs synthesize and secrete this immunoglobulin, which is then linked to a small protein produced by the epithelial cells, called secretory piece, and the complex is secreted externally. Secretory IgA is important in local protection against tissue invasion by many pathogens. The role of serum IgA is conjectural; it is not a precursor for the secretory form.

The largest immunoglobulin is IgM (macroglobulin), with a molecular weight of approximately 900,000. This immunoglobulin usually constitutes the first detectable antibody that is synthesized following antigenic challenge. A sensitive relationship exists between the circulating levels of IgG and IgM antibodies. Specific IgM antibodies may facilitate the production of IgG antibodies; in turn, the latter serve to inhibit the further production of IgM. The levels of IgG antibodies generally rise to high concentrations and persist appreciably longer than those of the IgM class.

The two other classes of immunoglobulins are minor serum components. There is little information about the function of IgD; it is present in only minute quantities in normal blood. However, as discussed previously, it appears to be an important antigen receptor on certain B cells. IgE is responsible for allergic reactions. This immunoglobulin is able to bind and remain fixed to tissue mast cells (see page 57). Reaction between these antibodies and corresponding antigens (allergens) serves to induce the mast cell to release histamine and other mediators of the allergic response (see Table 11).

The structure of immunoglobulin molecules has been well defined (Fig. 30). Each unit consists of four polypeptide chains, two identical light chains (L chains) and two identical heavy chains (H chains). The four chains are held together by disulfide bonds. Light chains may be of two types, designated kappa (κ) or lambda (λ), and are common to all classes of immunoglobulins. In contrast, heavy chains are specific for each class of immunoglobulins and are named in accordance with the class. Thus, for IgG, IgA, IgM, IgD, and IgE, the heavy chains are designated respectively gamma (γ), alpha (α), mu (μ), delta (δ), and epsilon (ε). Each immunoglobulin consists of two identical heavy chains that determine the class of immunoglobulin and two identical light chains that may be either type kappa or lambda.

Each immunoglobulin unit contains two antigen combining sites. Antigenic specificity is determined by the amino acid sequence of the N terminal end of both the light and the heavy chains; thus both chains contribute to the structure of the binding site. The portion of each chain that is specifically modified to react with the antigen is designated the "variable region"; the remainder is called the "constant" region. The antigen-reactive portion of the immunoglobulin

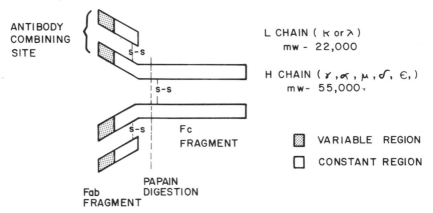

ANTIBODY COMBINING SITE

L CHAIN (κ or λ)
mw - 22,000

H CHAIN (γ, α, μ, δ, ε,)
mw - 55,000.

Fc FRAGMENT

▨ VARIABLE REGION

☐ CONSTANT REGION

Fab FRAGMENT

PAPAIN DIGESTION

FIGURE 30. Structure of the basic immunoglobulin subunit. Each subunit has two antibody combining sites. The Fc portion of the molecule is responsible for several activities, some of which are indicated on the diagram.

molecule is unique for each clone of antibodies; this portion has been termed the *idiotype.*

The digestion products of the immunoglobulin molecule after papain treatment are often used to designate specific regions. Papain splits the molecule into three pieces: two identical Fab fragments composed of the light chains and the corresponding portions of the heavy chains, and the Fc portion composed of the two terminal ends of the heavy chains. The Fc portion has important functions; it determines properties such as complement fixation, skin fixation, binding to cells, and placental transfer.

The same basic structure is common to all immunoglobulins. IgG, IgD, and IgE are monomers of this unit. Serum IgA may exist as either a monomer or a dimer. In molecules containing two or more subunits, the components are bound together by a polypeptide known as the J chain. Serum IgM consists of five monomeric units bound together by J chains into one molecule. Thus, this immunoglobulin has 10 potential antibody combining sites. Secretory IgA is believed to consist of IgA molecules that are held together by an additional piece, secretory piece, which is produced by epithelial cells of the mucosa.

The serum concentration of each class of immunoglobulin is determined by several factors: the rate of synthesis, the rate of elimination, and the distribution of immunoglobulin between the extravascular and intravascular fluids. IgG, which is present in the highest concentration, has the longest life span, 23 days, while both IgD and IgE are eliminated rapidly with a half life of less than 3 days. Almost half of IgG and IgA is intravascular; the remainder is present in the extravascular spaces. By contrast, IgM, because of its large molecular size, does not escape from the vascular system in any significant amount; therefore, more than 80 percent is intravascular. Except in situations such as the nephrotic syndrome in which there is a "glomerular leak," virtually no immunoglobulins are found in the urine.

In an immunoglobulin-synthesizing plasma cell, the light and heavy chains are produced separately on different cytoplasmic polyribosomes. The rate-limiting factor in the production of antibody is the synthesis of the heavy chains. Light chains will combine rapidly with heavy chains as the latter are formed, yielding a complete immunoglobulin molecule. In normal individuals, a balance exists between the production of light and heavy chains so that there is virtually no excess of light chains. However, in malignant diseases involving the plasma cells, light chains may be synthesized in marked excess or, in some cases, only light chains are produced. Free light chains are rapidly filtered from the serum by the renal glomeruli, producing a monoclonal "spike" on urine electrophoresis. This is sometimes referred to as Bence Jones proteinuria (see page 92).

Analysis of Serum Proteins

Serum protein electrophoresis serves as the major clinical tool for detecting immunoglobulin abnormalities. This method of separation is based on the net electrical charge of serum proteins. Most of the immunoglobulins reside in the gammaglobulin region; this is the slowest anodal migrating fraction. Thus, the term gammaglobulin has been used synonymously with immunoglobulins. However, the two are not identical, as some antibodies migrate more rapidly and will be found in the beta or the alpha$_2$ regions.

Three types of alterations in immunoglobulins can be identified by serum electrophoresis: (1) *hypogammaglobulinemia,* a reduction in the total quantity of immunoglobulins, (2) *polyclonal gammopathy,* a diffuse or heterogeneous increase in many antibody species, and (3) *monoclonal gammopathy,* the presence of an excess amount of a single homogeneous immunoglobulin. The last entity is composed of a single type of light chain and one type of heavy chain. Monoclonal immunoglobulins are seen characteristically in multiple myeloma and macroglobulinemia. On electrophoresis, the single protein species appears as a tall, narrow-based "spike." In contrast, polyclonal gammopathies result in a broad-based, rounded, irregular peak; these are found in many infections and diffuse inflammatory conditions. Polyclonal gammopathies contain a mixture of different antibody species; thus, they contain both lambda and kappa light chains and several different types of heavy chains. Examples of the different electrophoretic patterns are shown in Figure 31.

Although serum electrophoresis provides an adequate screening procedure, it does not distinguish among the various types of immunoglobulins. For example, by serum electrophoresis, a monoclonal gammopathy cannot be identified as IgG, IgA, IgM, IgD, or IgE abnormality. Also, it may not detect a deficiency in one type of immunoglobulin in the presence of normal or increased levels of others. More specific determination requires immunoelectrophoresis (IEP), a highly sensitive technique that can identify qualitative immunoglobulin abnormalities. IEP, however, is not a technique useful for quantitating immunoglobulins. Routinely, the amounts of a monoclonal immunoglobulin are followed by serial serum electrophoresis.

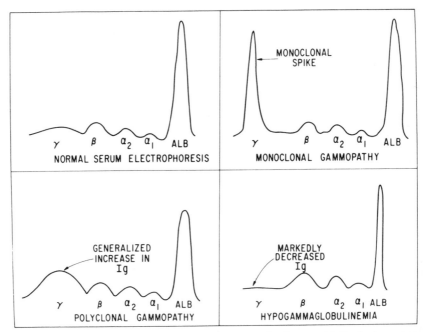

FIGURE 31. Serum protein electrophoretic patterns. As discussed in the text, a monoclonal "spike" represents the overproduction of a single species of antibody; a polyclonal pattern is seen when there are excessive amounts of multiple types of antibodies.

LYMPHOCYTE DISORDERS

Lymphocytosis and Lymphopenia

In most normal individuals, the blood lymphocyte count ranges from 1,500 to 4,000 cells per mm³ (see Table 1). Lymphopenia, a decrease in the number of circulating cells, is seen in both normal individuals and a variety of pathologic processes (Table 12). Certain apparently "normal" individuals show a consistent reduction in circulating lymphocytes; the basis for this finding is unidentified and, by itself, does not represent a "cause of alarm." However, lymphopenia is also seen in association with a number of infectious, neoplastic, and connective tissue diseases. Transient reductions routinely accompany many "stressful" or acute inflammatory conditions, including acute viral or bacterial infections. Furthermore, in many chronic infections, such as tuberculosis, lymphopenia is observed commonly.

   Patients with disseminated neoplasms often show a reduced number of circulating lymphocytes. In some neoplasms, such as carcinoma of the breast or stomach, low lymphocyte counts are a poor prognostic sign. By contrast, in

TABLE 12. Causes of Lymphopenia and Lymphocytosis

Lymphopenia (<1500/mm³)
1. No apparent disease.
2. Acute inflammatory disorders.
3. Corticosteroids.
4. Immune deficiency diseases.
5. Chronic infections.
6. Neoplasms.
7. Connective tissue diseases.

Lymphocytosis (>4000/mm³)
1. Infectious mononucleosis and related diseases.
2. Pertussis (whopping cough).
3. Lymphoid malignancies.
   a. Chronic lymphocytic leukemia.
   b. Leukemic phase of lymphomas.
   c. Acute lymphoblastic leukemia.

patients with Hodgkin's disease, lymphopenia may occur with apparently minimal tumor burden and does not necessarily indicate a poor prognosis. Reduced blood lymphocyte counts also are observed frequently in patients with diffuse connective tissue diseases, particularly systemic lupus erythematosus (SLE). In these patients, the lymphocyte reduction may result from the presence of antilymphocytic antibodies which cause an autoimmune destruction of these cells.

Lymphopenia may also occur as the result of therapy for various diseases. Cytotoxic drugs and irradiation cause lymphopenia; in some cases, radiation-induced lymphopenia may be of prolonged duration. Another agent that preferentially affects peripheral lymphocytes is corticosteroids. In certain species, such as the mouse, rat, and rabbit, steroids cause rapid lympholysis. However, in man and several other species (guinea pigs, monkeys), steroids are not primarily lympholytic; rather, they cause a rapid decrease in the blood lymphocyte count due to cell sequestration in tissues, particularly the bone marrow. Steroid effects are maximal four hours after intravenous injection; by 24 hours the effects are reversed, and the blood lymphocyte count has returned to normal.

Lymphocytosis is rarely encountered in normal individuals. The most common causes of blood lymphocyte counts in excess of 4,000 per mm³ are certain viral infections, such as infectious mononucleosis, and neoplasms of the lymphoid systems. In mononucleosis, many of the circulating lymphocytes have an atypical appearance; these cells are T lymphocytes that are transformed in response to the Epstein-Barr virus (EBV), the infecting agent. The virus itself is not found in T cells; it only infects B lymphocytes.

An increased number of blood lympocytes with morphologic changes similar to those found in infectious mononucleosis is seen in other diseases such as those due to cytomegalovirus, viral hepatitis, and toxoplasmosis. In these diseases, the total lymphocyte count is often normal or only slightly increased. One infectious disease, pertussis (whopping cough), is often associated with a very high blood lymphocyte count. Unlike mononucleosis, the lymphocytes seen in patients with pertussis are small, normal-appearing cells. It appears that these bacteria mobilize lymphocytes from peripheral lymphoid tissues.

Lymphocytosis is also seen in neoplasms affecting the lymphoid system. Chronic lymphocytic leukemia is characterized by persistent elevations of the blood lymphocyte count; most of the circulating cells appear to be small lymphocytes without cytologic abnormalities. Increased blood lymphocyte counts may also occur as part of non-Hodgkin's lymphoma. Lymphoblasts are the characteristic cells present in the circulation of patients with acute lymphoblastic leukemia.

Immune Deficiency Diseases

Disorders characterized by reduced ability to mount immune responses are subdivided into two groups: (1) those associated with an underlying pathologic process (secondary immune deficiency states) and (2) those in which there is no other defect present (primary immune deficiency disorders). Within each group, defects may be categorized by the major manifestations: failure of humoral antibody formation (hypogammaglobulinemia), deficient cellular immunity, or combined failure of both defense mechanisms.

PRIMARY IMMUNE DEFICIENCY DISEASES

The division of peripheral lymphocytes into two populations, each responsible for a different type of immunity, lends itself to the model of immune deficiencies shown in Figure 32. Abnormalities may involve the common immunologic stem cell, thus causing defects in both types of immune responses, or an isolated abnormality in either T- or B-cell populations. A brief description of these disorders is included below.

Among the inherited disorders, *severe combined immunodeficiency* (SCID) represents the most severe form of immunologic failure. Several different forms have been recognized, including an inherited deficiency in the enzyme ADA (see page 79). Manifestations are usually apparent within the first few months of life; they include recurrent infections, frequently with organisms of low pathogenicity, severe diarrhea, chronic skin rashes, a profound failure to thrive, and death usually within the first year of life. As would be expected from the nature of the defect, laboratory studies indicate a marked reduction in all types of immunoglobulins, decreased numbers of lymphocytes in the blood and in the peripheral tissues, and an absence of cellular and humoral responses to test antigens. Immunologic reconstitution has been achieved with bone marrow transplants from HLA-compatible donors.

DiGeorge's syndrome results from a failure of embryologic development of the third and fourth branchial pouches and therefore results in a congenital absence of both the thymus and parathyroids. The immunologic defects appear early in life, usually within the first few months after birth, and may be associated with hypocalcemic tetany (due to the parathyroid abnormality). Clinical manifestations of the immune disorder are similar to those seen in SCID; most frequently,

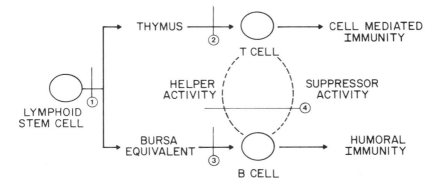

① SEVERE COMBINED IMMUNODEFICIENCY DISEASE (SCID)
② DI GEORGE SYNDROME
③ X-LINKED AGAMMAGLOBULINEMIA
④ COMMON VARIABLE HYPOGAMMAGLOBULINEMIA (CVH)

FIGURE 32. Several immunodeficiency diseases can be viewed as cellular blocks in the normal maturation of lymphocytes. In addition, many cases of common variable hypogammaglobulinemia appear to result from excessive T suppressor activity.

affected children die within the first year of life. Laboratory findings include a decreased number of T lymphocytes in the blood and the thymic-dependent regions of peripheral tissues. By contrast, B lymphocytes are present and appear to function normally. Immunologic testing reveals an absence of cell-mediated immune responses. By contrast, immunoglobulin levels may be near normal, and these individuals show normal humoral antibody responses to thymic-independent antigens. As expected, they do not respond well to thymic-dependent challenges. Some of these patients have been treated successfully with thymic grafts. As described previously, patients deficient in the enzyme PNP (see page 79) also show a selective failure in T-cell immunity.

X-linked agammaglobulinemia is inherited as a sex-linked recessive disorder. Characteristically, affected boys develop recurrent respiratory and skin infections; the disease-causing organisms are primarily the extracellular, catalase-negative pyogenic bacteria (pneumococci, meningococci, streptococci, and *H. influenzae*). Agammaglobulinemic children respond to most viral infections in a manner similar to normal individuals. Laboratory data include a normal number of circulating lymphocytes and intact responses in tests for cellular immunity, but extremely low levels of immunoglobulins and no increase in antibody titers following challenges with specific antigens. Histologic examination of lymphatic tissues shows that the thymic-independent regions are poorly developed, and plasma cells are absent. In most, there is a marked deficiency in the number of B cells in the peripheral blood; by contrast, T cells are normal. Unlike disorders affecting cellular immunity, these individuals can survive into adult life with appropriate treatment (antibiotics and replacement gammaglobulin).

Common variable hypogammaglobulinemia (CVH) is a heterogeneous group of disorders characterized by reduced serum immunoglobulin levels; these appear after a period of apparently normal production. The syndrome can occur at any age, and both sexes are affected equally. The clinical manifestations tend to be highly variable. In part, they reflect the severity of the hypogammaglobulinemia. Patients with very low levels of immunoglobulins are prone to recurrent infections due to encapsulated bacteria. Cell-mediated immunity is either normal or only slightly impaired; these individuals are not prone to infections by intracellular organisms. Other complications of CVH include a wide variety of autoimmune disorders, including immunologically-related blood dyscrasias. The pathogenesis of this syndrome is highly variable. In some patients, B lymphocytes are absent. Others show a normal number of B cells, but these cells are defective in that they are unable to proliferate or mature into plasma cells. In other patients, the primary abnormality leading to hypogammaglobulinemia appears to be a lack of T helper cells. Perhaps the most common cause of CVH is abnormal T suppressor cells that act to prevent normal humoral antibody responses. Patients with this form of CVH have circulating B cells which, when separated from T cells, are capable of normal immunoglobulin synthesis *in vitro*. However, the isolated T cells suppress immunoglobulin production by both autologous and allogeneic B cells.

Selective absence of IgA is the most common of the primary deficiencies; it occurs in approximately 1 in 600 individuals. They lack IgA in both the serum and external secretions; by contrast, IgG and IgM levels are usually normal. Despite the lack of IgA, which is thought to be important for local protection at mucosal surfaces, the majority of these patients do not suffer from recurrent infections. Only about 20 percent of patients with this deficiency incur an increased number of infections; these occur primarily in the respiratory and/or gastrointestinal tract. It appears that in most IgA-deficient subjects, mucosal immunity is maintained by other immunoglobulins. Although not prone to infection, these IgA-deficient patients experience an abnormally high incidence of autoimmune and allergic disorders. Lymphocyte studies indicate that almost all affected patients have IgA-bearing B lymphocytes in their blood. The differentiation of these cells into IgA-secreting plasma cells, however, is blocked. An abnormality in the T helper cell population may be responsible for this maturation defect.

SECONDARY IMMUNE DEFICIENCIES

Immune deficiencies occur often during the course of many acute and chronic diseases. In fact, there is increasing awareness that failure to maintain immune homeostasis is a major cause of morbidity and mortality. In addition, the widespread use of drugs capable of suppressing immune responses serves as an additional cause of deficiency states. Although detailed discussions of each of these entities is not possible, it is important to recognize that virtually any *severely ill patient* may have compromised immune defenses; the most immediate consequence of these abnormalities will be an increased risk of infection.

Malignancies involving lymphocytes are common causes of immune deficiencies. Furthermore, characteristics of the malignant cell can often be related to the immunodeficiency.

B-cell malignancies are a common cause of immune deficiency. In parallel with the normal maturation of B lymphocytes, each stage of development has a malignant counterpart (Fig. 33). The cells in many cases of ALL show characteristics of either immature B lymphocytes or pre-B cells. Chronic lymphocytic leukemia (CLL) and well-differentiated lymphoid lymphomas appear to arise from mature, small B cells. Waldenstrom's macroglobulinemia simulates the early stages of B-cell activation by antigen, and multiple myeloma is the malignant counterpart of the differentiated plasma cell stage. With the exception of the acute leukemias, all of these diseases are characterized by prominent abnormalities in immunoglobulin production. CLL patients frequently develop hypogammaglobulinemia; macroglobulinemia is characterized by overproduction of monoclonal IgM, and multiple myeloma by monoclonal immunoglobulin (G, A, D, or rarely E) and/or a portion of the immunoglobulin (monoclonal light chains). In the last two diseases, the patients frequently have reduced synthesis of normal polyclonal immunoglobulins; thus, they are "functionally" hypogammaglobulinemic. Cell-mediated immunity in the B-cell neoplasms is usually normal or only mildly impaired.

Acute lymphoblastic leukemia (ALL) is the most common form of leukemia in children; clinical features are discussed on page 23. Phenotypic studies of patients with ALL indicate that the blasts in 60 to 80 percent of the cases are considered to be null lymphocytes (non-T non-B cells). Only 5 percent have features of B cells (sIg$^+$), while 10 to 20 percent are considered to be of T-cell origin. Of note, approximately 20 percent of the null-cell leukemias are found to be pre-B cells. These blasts show scant amounts of cytoplasmic IgM but lack detectable surface immunoglobulins. In addition, genetic analysis suggests that many of the "so called" true null cells are, in fact, in the B-cell lineage. Patients with early ALL do not show prominent immunologic abnormalities primarily because affected individuals retain a nearly normal complement of more mature cells.

Chronic lymphocytic leukemia is a disorder, usually of the elderly, characterized by a slow but progressive increase in the number of morphologically-normal, small lymphocytes in the blood. It is not unusual for the absolute lymphocyte count to exceed 100,000 per mm^3. In addition to lymphocytosis, patients with CLL will often show lymphadenopathy, hepatosplenomegaly, and lymphocytic infiltration in the marrow. The disease tends to run a relatively benign course; the median survival is six to eight years, and it is not unusual for patients to survive 15 years or longer. By immunofluorescent techniques, leukemic cells in most patients have the phenotypic characteristics of normal B cells (e.g., sIg$^+$). The most common immunologic abnormality is an impairment in humoral antibody responses. A high percentage (in some series, 40 to 60 percent) of patients develop panhypogammaglobulinemia, and, by quantitating individual immunoglobulins, virtually all patients show decreased levels of one

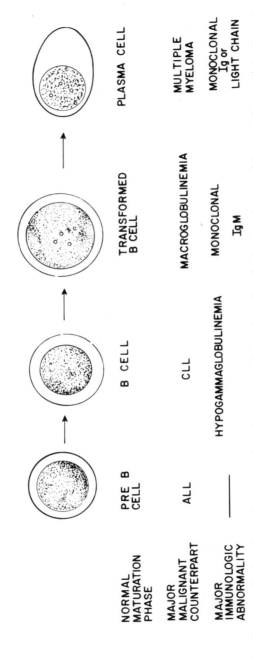

FIGURE 33. B-cell malignancies can be viewed as a neoplastic transformation of cells at each stage of the normal maturation sequence. Furthermore, in most disorders, there is a corresponding immunologic abnormality affecting the B cell system (i.e., hypogammaglobulinemia and/or production of a monoclonal antibody).

or more types. The reduced levels of immunoglobulins in these patients result from decreased production of humoral antibodies rather than from an increased catabolic rate. Even those patients with normal levels of immunoglobulins may show defects in responding to certain immunologic stimuli, particularly those classified as primary responses. CLL patients are particularly susceptible to infections by encapsulated pyogenic bacteria; recurrent pneumococcal pneumonia and septicemia constitute a major cause of morbidity and mortality. In contrast to the profound defect in humoral antibody responses, parameters of cellular immunity tend to be relatively normal.

In addition to the defect of immunoglobulin production, there is an increased incidence of "autoimmune disorders" in patients with CLL. Malignant B lymphocytes may elaborate humoral antibodies that react with antigens on the patient's own cells. Alternatively, an imbalance in normal, residual lymphocyte populations may result in a breakdown of normal self-recognition. Regardless of the mechanisms, these autoantibodies are often directed at one or more of the formed elements of the blood and can result in autoimmune hemolytic anemia, immune thrombocytopenia, and/or immune neutropenia. Recent studies suggest that both the impaired antibody production and the loss of normal tolerance mechanisms may result in part from defective T-cell regulation.

Multiple myeloma is a disorder in which there is a neoplastic production of a single clone of plasma cells; these cells elaborate a homogeneous immunoglobulin and/or single type of free light chain. Myeloma, like CLL, is a disease of the elderly and is characterized by three major features: (1) the infiltration of the marrow by an abnormal number of plasma cells, (2) the presence of a monoclonal immunoglobulin spike in the serum and/or a single type of free light chain in the urine, and (3) less frequently, the appearance of characteristic "punched out" osteolytic lesions on x-ray films of bones; these are due to localized plasma cell proliferation with resultant bone destruction secondary to elaboration of substances such as osteoclast-activating factor.

Although the malignant cell in myeloma is a plasma cell, idiotypic identification of myeloma proteins indicates that excess numbers of pre-B cells contain the same antibody determinants. This suggests that the neoplasm may actually arise in a cell early in the maturation sequence; this cell retains the property of differentiation but is not susceptible to normal regulatory mechanisms.

Depending on the relative quantities of light and heavy chains synthesized by the malignant clone of plasma cells, the monoclonal protein manifests itself as a complete immunoglobulin, free light chains, or both. Thus, three distinct types of protein abnormalities can be recognized (Table 13). In the first, the

TABLE 13. Protein Abnormalities in Multiple Myeloma

COMPARATIVE SYNTHESIS OF HEAVY AND LIGHT CHAINS	MONOCLONAL ABNORMALITIES	
	SERUM	URINE
$H = L$	+	0
$H < L$	+	+
L only	0	+

abnormal clone elaborates equal quantities of one type of light chain and one type of heavy chain; these are assembled into a single homogeneous immunoglobulin that is secreted into the circulation. As a result, there is a monoclonal spike on serum electrophoresis; the urine does not show free light chains. In the second grouping, the abnormal clone is able to produce both heavy and light chains, but there is excessive production of the latter. Available heavy chains are incorporated into complete immunoglobulin molecules which produce a monoclonal serum spike. The excess free light chains are cleared rapidly and completely from the circulation by the kidneys. These can be identified as a monoclonal protein in the urine. In the third grouping, the malignant plasma cells produce a homogeneous light chain without a corresponding heavy chain. As a result, the serum will not show a monoclonal spike, but the free light chains can be identified readily in the urine as a spike on urinary electrophoresis. Free light chains in the urine are also called Bence Jones protein.

It appears that for any single patient, the quantity of the monoclonal protein is directly proportional to the total number of malignant cells. Thus, serial measures of the monoclonal protein by serum electrophoresis provide the most accurate means of assessing progression of the disease or responses to therapy. In general, a 50 percent change in concentration is considered significant.

In addition to the production of an abnormal quantity of a particular immunoglobulin, patients with multiple myeloma commonly show a marked reduction in the production of normal immunoglobulins. As a result, these patients display the same spectrum of increased susceptibility to infections as observed in CLL. The basis for the defect in antibody production is not defined fully—it may be the result of excessive suppression of normal antibody synthesis by either macrophages or T lymphocytes.

A major feature of myeloma is renal failure; this is the cause of death of approximately one third of affected patients. Many factors can contribute to the pathogenesis of renal failure. The major cause, however, appears to be related to the presence of free light chains in the tubules. These chains are filtered and can be reabsorbed by renal tubular cells. However, the tubular cells are unable to degrade these polypeptides properly; this leads ultimately to tubular cell death, a fibrotic reaction, and renal failure. It should be noted that the presence of light chains in the urine alone does not necessarily indicate the patient will develop renal failure. Why some patients can handle light chains without problems while others develop severe renal failure is not known.

Macroglobulinemia is a form of malignant lymphoma characterized by excessive production of monoclonal IgM. The neoplastic cells have features of both lymphocytes and plasma cells, hence, the designation lymphocytoid plasma cells. Immunologically, they appear as transitional cells and are both sIg$^+$ and cIg$^+$. The major clinical features of this disease are dominated by evidence of a lymphoid malignancy (lymphadenopathy, hepatosplenomegaly, bone marrow infiltration by neoplastic cells) and the presence of large quantities of serum IgM leading to the hyperviscosity syndrome. Many manifestations of this syndrome result from decreased blood flow and include central nervous system abnormalities (ranging from mild headache and/or focal neurologic defects to coma and convulsions), cardiopulmonary failure (as evidenced by congestive heart failure, coronary artery disease, or respiratory insufficiency), ocular abnormalities, and a bleeding diathesis. Because most IgM is intravascular, temporary improvement in the hyperviscosity syndrome can be achieved rapidly by plasma exchange.

Monoclonal gammopathies of undetermined origin (also called benign monoclonal gammopathies) are now being discovered incidentally in many patients due to the widespread application of protein studies in clinical medicine. The majority of these individuals are elderly and, despite careful evaluation, do not show any clinical evidence of a B-cell malignancy. Furthermore, prolonged follow-up of these individuals indicates that the monoclonal protein often remains stable, and other features suggestive of myeloma do not become apparent. Only a small fraction of these patients ultimately develop myeloma or other B-cell malignancies; in these, the evolution to an overt malignant state often requires several years. At present, it is not possible to predict accurately which patients will progress to a B-cell malignancy. Thus, all patients with undefined monoclonal gammopathies require careful follow-up with particular attention to changes in the quantity of monoclonal proteins.

Lymphoid (non-Hodgkin's) lymphomas comprise a heterogeneous group of malignancies. The clinical manifestations include lymphadenopathy, hepatosplenomegaly, and bone marrow involvement. Patients frequently experience a variety of symptoms including night sweats, fevers, and weight loss. This disease can occur in any stage of life, but the frequency increases with age.

The diagnosis of a non-Hodgkin's lymphoma is made by biopsy of an involved organ. In addition, the histologic characteristics of the tumor have proved to be a prime determinant of prognosis. Although several classifications of these tumors have been proposed, none has proved to be clearly superior. At present, the Rapapport classification is the most widely used system. Based on the pattern of infiltration into an involved node, diseases are subdivided into diffuse or nodular groups. They are further categorized as to the degree of differentiation of the malignant cells. Five cellular types are recognized: well-differentiated lymphocytic, poorly-differentiated lymphocytic, histiocytic, mixed lymphocytic and histiocytic, and undifferentiated. The term "histiocytic" lymphoma is a misnomer; most of these neoplasms appear to be of lymphocytic origin. This system and the other classifications appear to be most valuable in that they provide a measure of the aggressiveness of the tumor and, in turn, the average survival. For each cellular stage, nodular disease tends to have a better prognosis than the corresponding diffuse form. Likewise, as the cells become more differentiated, survival improves. Thus, untreated patients with well-differentiated lymphocytic lymphoma have a median survival of more than nine years while that for patients with diffuse poorly-differentiated lymphocytic disease is less than one year.

The vast majority of non-Hodgkin's lymphomas are of B-cell origin. (A typical survey indicates that 68 percent of these tumors are derived from B cells, 19 percent from T cells, 13 percent are undefined, and only 0.2 percent are of myeloid origin and thus truly histiocytic). The relationship between the

TABLE 14. Lymphocytic Lymphoma

HISTOLOGIC CLASSIFICATION	CELL TYPE
A. *Nodular*	
1. Lymphocytic	*All* are B-cell tumors
Well differentiated	
2. Lymphocytic	
Poorly differentiated (? arise from germinal center cells)	
3. Mixed	
Lymphocytic—histiocytic	
4. Histiocytic	
B. *Diffuse*	
1. Lymphocytic	50–60% B cells
Well differentiated	33% unclassified
2. Lymphocytic	5–10% T cells
Poorly differentiated	5% myeloloid
3. Mixed	
Lymphocytic—histiocytic	
4. Histiocytic	
5. Undifferentiated	
6. Lymphoblastic	

histiologic and immunologic classifications of non-Hodgkin's lymphomas is shown in Table 14. Although most malignant cells in non-Hodgkin's lymphomas are of immunologic origin, immune abnormalities are generally not pronounced. However, some patients do show monoclonal serum immunoglobulins; others may express autoimmune phenomena or manifest a humoral immune deficiency.

The spread of non-Hodgkin's lymphoma can be related to the cell type. Well-differentiated neoplastic lymphocytes have the capacity to recirculate; thus dissemination tends to occur early in the course of the disease. Almost all patients have widespread involvement at the time of presentation. With these tumors, the pathways for cell migration resemble closely those of normal cells. In addition, the malignant cells appear to have a slow rate of turnover; in total, their kinetic and circulatory activities are similar to those of normal, long-lived recirculating B cells.

As the cell assumes a more malignant cytologic appearance, it shows a reduced tendency to migrate via physiologic pathways. The most malignant forms generally spread from their site of origin only by pathologic migration, either through the lymphatic system or hematogenously. These tumors metastasize in a manner similar to nonlymphoid malignancies.

The management of patients with non-Hodgkin's lymphoma depends upon both the histologic stage and its anatomic spread. The highly malignant forms may present as localized tumors; with these, radiation therapy may be curative. However, 85 to 90 percent of patients with non-Hodgkin's lymphoma have disseminated disease at the time of presentation. In patients with highly malignant variants, increased survival can be achieved frequently with aggressive chemotherapy. However, this beneficial response depends on achieving a total disappearance of all evidence of disease, a complete remission. By contrast, there are little data indicating that survival in the well-differentiated forms is influenced by therapy.

T-cell lymphomas, in general, are less common and consequently less well-defined than their B-cell counterparts. Approximately 15 to 20 percent of the acute lymphoblastic leukemias are of T-cell origin. Compared with the null-cell variants, T-cell ALL tends to occur in older children, is often associated with a mediastinal mass, responds less satisfactorily to chemotherapy, and has a poorer prognosis. A closely-related disorder, T lymphoblastic lymphoma is an aggressive neoplasm presenting usually as a mediastinal tumor. In more than half of these patients, leukemic transformation to T-cell ALL occurs during the course of the disease. The prognosis of lymphoblastic lymphoma is very poor. Likewise, rare cases of CLL are of T-cell origin.

The most well-defined neoplasms of the T cell system are the cutaneous lymphomas, mycosis fungoides—Sezary syndrome. This disease is a chronic, slowly progressive neoplasm involving primarily the skin. Only late in the course of the disease is there extensive neoplastic infiltration in lymph nodes and visceral organs. Mycosis fungoides usually presents as a polymorphic skin eruption that often resembles eczema or psoriasis. Later, it progresses to a plaque-like stage; the third stage is characterized by cutaneous tumors and ulcerating lesions. Lymphadenopathy and visceral involvement occur during this stage. Sezary syndrome represents a "leukemic" phase of mycosis fungoides in which significant numbers of the neoplastic lymphocytes are in the blood. Furthermore, generalized erythroderma usually is present. The principal source of the abnormal blood cells appears to be the skin tumors. Immunologically, the neoplastic cells infiltrating the skin and the atypical lymphocytes in the blood are of T-cell origin. They belong primarily to the T helper subset. Morphologically, the nuclei of these cells are fairly distinctive in appearance. Electromicroscopic examination shows the nuclei of the cells to have very dense repetitive clefting such that they are said to be "cerebriform."

HODGKIN'S DISEASE

This is a malignant lymphoma that has unique immunologic and lymphocytic features. In this disease, the primary sites of involvement are lymph nodes. Histologically, they are characterized by the presence of Reed-Sternberg cells, multinucleated cells that appear to be of macrophage origin (see page 24).

One feature of this disease that is of considerable interest is the direct correlation between the lymphocytic infiltration in the involved tissues and survival. Those tumors that display large numbers of lymphocytes (the lymphocyte-predominant form) tend to have the best prognosis; by contrast, the more malignant variants (mixed cellularity and lymphocyte-depleted) show reduced numbers of lymphocytes in affected tissues. These neoplasms tend to disseminate early, and such patients have a much shorter survival. The correlation between lymphocytic infiltration and aggressiveness of the tumor suggests that the lymphoid cells constitute an important host defense mechanism that serves to limit the progression of this disease.

A second feature of note is the association between Hodgkin's disease and cell-mediated immune defects. Many patients, including those with early and asymptomatic disease, show abnormalities such as lymphopenia, decreased lymphocyte responses to mitogens, and cutaneous anergy. It appears that there are multiple factors that cause these abnormalities, one of which is the presence of suppressor macrophages. These phagocytes may act by synthesizing excess amounts of inhibitory prostaglandins. There is an imprecise correlation between cell-mediated immune abnormalities and either histologic staging or anatomic dissemination. However, defects tend to be more common in patients with advanced disease. Most of these abnormalities will be reversed if the malignancy is treated successfully. This suggests that the immune defects are probably due to the disease itself, rather than an underlying abnormality predisposing to malignant transformation. Nevertheless, the abnormalities in cellular immunity appear to be a predisposing factor leading to increased susceptibility to infections with intracellular pathogens.

IMMUNOGENETICS

In recent years, there has been increasing awareness of important genetic determinants that affect immune responses. The predominant influences are exerted by the major histocompatibility complex (MHC) which, in man, is located on chromosome #6. In man, this complex is termed the *human leukocyte antigen (HLA)* system. Genes in this complex are of prime importance in determining self-recognition and in regulating many immune responses to exogenous antigens. Furthermore, it appears to be a major factor contributing to the susceptibility to certain diseases (e.g., susceptibility to ankylosing spondylitis is closely linked to the presence of the HLA B27 antigen). There are four well-defined regions (loci) within the HLA complex; these are designated the A, B, C, and D/Dr regions (Fig. 34). Each locus has between 8 and 39 alleles, which accounts readily for the great diversity of HLA types found in the general population.

Products of the A, B, and C loci are defined by serologic tests; these antigens are found on all nucleated cells and platelets. The D/Dr locus is recognized both by the mixed lymphocyte culture assay and by serologic techniques.

CHROMOSOME # 6

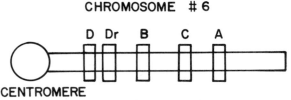

FIGURE 34. The arrangement of human histocompatability loci on chromosome #6.

Whether the two techniques measure identical or extremely close loci is still not determined. These antigens have a more restrictive expression; they are found in B cells, pre-B cells, monocytes, epithelial cells, and activated T cells, but are absent from resting T cells and plasma cells. The Dr antigens in man, like the Ia antigens in the mouse, are important in controlling cellular interactions among T cells, B cells, and macrophages, and in effecting certain cytotoxic reactions. For example, in order for sensitized lymphocytes to lyse virally-infected cells, there must be homology at the Dr locus between the killer and target cells. In addition, differences in alleles at the Dr locus provide the major stimulus for reactivity in a mixed-leukocyte culture assay (see page 77). It is of note that genes within the HLA complex are the loci controlling the synthesis of three complement components (C2, C4, and factor B).

As all four loci reside on a single chromosome, this unit is referred to as a *haplotype.* Each sibling receives one haplotype from each parent; thus, on a statistical basis, there is a 25 percent chance that two siblings will have identical HLA haplotypes. By contrast, the diversity in alleles at each locus indicates that it is extremely unlikely that unrelated individuals would match at all HLA loci. Exact matching of HLA antigens has proved extremely important in bone marrow transplants. Unless all HLA antigens are matched, the patient usually develops either graft rejection or fatal graft-versus-host disease.

BIBLIOGRAPHY

GENERAL:

KARNOVSKY ML AND BOLIS L: *Phagocytosis—Past and Future.* Academic Press, New York, 1982.

WINTROBE MM, JEE GR, BOGGS DR, BITHEL TC, FOERSTER J, ATHENS JW, AND JUKENS JN: *Clinical Hematology,* ed. 8. Lea & Febiger, Philadelphia, 1981.

MARROW STRUCTURE:

DEBRUYN PPH: *Structural substrates of bone marrow function.* Semin Hematol 18(3):179–193, 1981.

CELLULAR COOPERATION:

UNANUE ER: *Cooperation between mononuclear phagocytes and lymphocytes in immunity.* New Engl J Med 303(17):997–985, 1980.

HEMATOPOIETIC STEM CELLS:

FIALKOW P: *Clonal development and stem cell origin of proliferative disorders.* In Wyngarden and Smith (eds): *Cecil's Textbook of Medicine.* WB Saunders, Philadelphia, 1982, pp viii–121.

NEUTROPHILS:

BOGGS DR: *The kinetics of neutrophilic leukocytes in health and in disease.* Semin Hematol 4:359,1967.

Boggs DR: *The leukopenic state.* In Wyngarden and Smith (eds): *Cecil's Textbook of Medicine.* WB Saunders, Philadelphia, 1982, pp viii–119.

Holmes B, Quie PG, Windhorst DB, and Good RA: *Fatal granulomatous disease of childhood: An inborn abnormality of phagocytic function.* Lancet 1:1225, 1966.

Craddock PR, Hammerschmidt DE, Moldow CF, Yamada O, and Jacob HS: *Granulocyte aggregation as a manifestation of membrane interactions with complement—Possible role in leukocyte margination, microvascular occlusion, and endothelial damage.* Semin Hematol 16(2):140, 1979.

Schiffmann E, and Gallin JI: *Biochemistry of phagocyte chemotaxis.* In Horecker and Stadtman (eds): *Current Topics in Cellular Regulation, vol 15.* Academic Press, New York, 1979, pp 203–261.

Gallin JI, Wright DG, Malech HL, Davis JM, Klempner MS, and Kirkpatrick CH: *Disorders of phagocyte chemotoxis.* Ann Intern Med.92(4):520–538, 1980.

Harlan JM, Killen PD, Harker LA, Striker GE and Wright DG: *Neutrophil-mediated endothelial injury in vitro—Mechanisms of cell detachment.* J Clin Invest 68(6):1394–1403, 1981.

Snyderman R, and Goetzl EJ: *Molecular and cellular mechanisms of leukocyte chemotaxis.* Science 213:830–837, 1981.

Gabig TG, and Babiar BM: *The killing of pathogens by phagocytes.* Annu Rev Med 32:187, 1981.

Tauber AI: *Current views of neutrophil dysfunction. An integrated clinical perspective.* Am J Med 70:1237–1246, 1981.

Marx JL: *The leukotrienes in allergy and inflammation.* Science 215:1380–1383, 1982.

MONOCYTES AND MACROPHAGES:

Cline MJ, Lehrer RI, Territo MC, and Golde DW: *Monocytes and macrophages: Functions and diseases.* Ann Intern Med 88(1)78–88, 1978.

EOSINOPHILS:

Bass DA: *Behavior of eosinophils in acute inflammation.* J Clin Invest 56:870, 1975.

Butterworth AE, and David Jr: *Current concepts: Eosinophil function.* N Engl J Med 304(3):154–156, 1981.

McLaren DJ: *The role of eosinophils in tropical disease.* Semin Hematol 19(2):100–106, 1982.

BASOPHILS AND MAST CELLS:

Dvorak AM, and Dvorak HF: *Basophil—its morphology, biochemistry, motility, release reactions, recovery, and role in the inflammatory responses of IgE-mediated and cell-mediated origin.* Arch Pathol Lab Med 103(11):551, 1979.

WASSERMAN SI: *The mast cell and the inflammatory response.* In Pepys and Edwards (eds): *The Mast Cell.* University Park Press, Baltimore, 1979, pp 9–20.

LYMPHOCYTES—GENERAL:

KAY NE, ACKERMAN SK, AND DOUGLAS SD: *Anatomy of the immune system.* Semin Hematol 16:251, 1979.

WINKELSTEIN A, AND RABIN BS: *Lymphocyte biology.* Bull Rheum Dis 25:816, 1975.

WINKELSTEIN A: *The anatomy and physiology of lymphocytes.* In Lichtman (ed): *The Science and Practice of Clinical Medicine, vol 6. Hematology and Oncology.* Grune & Stratton, New York, 1980, p 165.

WINKELSTEIN A: *Lymphocytosis and lymphopenia.* In Lichtman (ed): *The Science and Practice of Clinical Medicine, vol 6. Hematology and Oncology.* Grune & Stratton, New York, 1980, p 168.

ZACHARSKI LR, AND LINMAN JW: *Lymphopenia: Its causes and significance.* Mayo Clin Proc 46:168, 1971.

LYMPHOCYTE SUBSETS:

BOWMAN WP, MELVIN S, AND MAUER AM: *Cell markers in lymphomas and leukemias.* Adv Intern Med 25:391, 1980.

BRODER S, MUUL L, MARSHALL S, ET AL: *Neoplasms of immunoregulatory T cells in clinical investigation.* J Invest Dermatol 74:267, 1980.

CANTOR, H, AND BOYSE EA: *Regulation of immune response by T-cell subclasses.* Contemp Top Immunol 7:47, 1977.

CHESS L, AND SCHLOSSMAN SF: *Human lymphocyte subpopulations.* Adv Immunol 25:213, 1977.

COOPER MD: *Pre-B cells: Normal and abnormal development.* J Clin Immunol 1:81, 1981.

GUPTA S, AND GOOD RA: *Markers of human lymphocyte subpopulations in primary immunodeficiency and lymphoproliferative disorders.* Semin Hematol 17:1, 1980.

KUNKEL HG: *Surface markers of human lymphocytes.* Johns Hopkins Med J 137:216, 1975.

MORETTA L, MINGARI MC, AND MORETTA A: *Human T-cell subpopulations in normal and pathologic conditions.* Immunol Rev 45:163, 1979.

NADLER LM, RITZ J, GRIFFIN JD ET AL: *Diagnosis and treatment of human leukemias and lymphomas utilizing monoclonal antibodies.* Prog Hematol 12:187, 1981.

REINHERZ EL, KUNG PC, GOLDSTEIN G, ET AL: *Separation of functional subsets of human T cells by a monoclonal antibody.* Proc Natl Acad Sci USA 76:4061, 1979.

REINHERZ EL, AND SCHLOSSMAN SF: *Regulation of immune response—Inducer and suppressor T-lymphocyte subsets in human beings.* N Engl J Med 303:370, 1980.

LYMPHOKINES:

COHEN S, MAYER M, PICK E, ET AL: *Current state of studies of mediators of cellular immunity: A progress report.* Cell Immunol 33:233, 1977.

ROCKLIN RE, BENDTZEN K, AND GREINEDER D: *Mediators of immunity: Lymphokines and monokines.* Adv Immunol 29:56, 1980.

RUSCETTI FW, AND GALLO RC: *Human T-lymphocyte growth factor: Regulation of growth and function of T lymphocytes.* Blood 57:379, 1981.

GLUCOCORTICOID EFFECTS:

FAUCI AS, DALE DC, AND BALOW JE: *Glucocorticosteroid therapy: Mechanisms of action and clinical considerations.* Ann Intern Med 84:304, 1976.

HAYNES BF, AND FAUCI AS: *The differential effect of in vivo hydrocortisone on the kinetics of subpopulations of human peripheral blood thymus-derived lymphocytes.* J Clin Invest 61:703, 1978.

CYTOTOXIC CELLS:

CEROTTINI JC, AND BRUNNER KT: *Cell-mediated cytotoxicity, allograft rejection and tumor immunity.* Adv Immunol 18:67, 1974.

HERBERMAN RB, DJEU JY, KAY HD, ORTALDO JR, RICCARDI C, BONNARD GD, ET AL: *Natural killer cells: Characteristics and regulation of activity.* Immunol Rev 44:43, 1979.

HERBERMAN RB, AND ORTALDO JR: *Natural killer cells: Their role in defenses against disease.* Science 214:24, 1981.

LOVCHIK JC, AND HONG R: *Antibody dependent cell-mediated cytolysis (ADCC): Analysis and projections.* Prog Allergy 22:1, 1977.

MACROPHAGES—LYMPHOCYTES INTERACTIONS:

CLINE MJ, LEHRER RI, TERRITO MC, ET AL: *Monocytes and macrophages: Functions and diseases.* Ann Intern Med 88:78, 1978.

MACKANESS GB: *The monocyte in cellular immunity.* Semin Hematol 7:172, 1970.

NORTH RJ: *The concept of the activated macrophage.* J Immunol 121:806, 1978.

ROSENTHAL AS: *Regulation of the immune response—Role of the macrophage.* New Engl J Med 303:1153, 1980.

UNANUE ER, AND ROSENTHAL AS (EDS): *Macrophage Regulation of Immunity.* Academic Press, New York, 1980.

WING EJ, AND REMINGTON JS: *Lymphocytes and macrophages in cell-mediated immunity.* In Mandell, Douglas, and Bennett (eds): *Principles and Practices of Infectious Diseases.* John Wiley & Sons, New York, 1979, p 83.

LYMPHOCYTE CIRCULATION:

FORD WL: *Lymphocyte migration and immune response.* Prog Allergy 19:1, 1975.

SPRENT J: *Recirculating lymphocytes.* In Marchalonis (ed): *The Lymphocyte: Structure and Function.* Marcel Dekker, New York, 1977, p 43.

CHO Y, AND DEBRUYN PH: *Transcellular migration of lymphocytes through the walls of the smooth-surfaced squamous endothelial venules in the lymph node: Evidence for the direct entry of lymphocytes into the blood circulation of the lymph node.* J Ultrastruct Res 74:259, 1981.

WEISSMAN IL, GUTMAN GA, AND FRIEDBERG SH: *Tissue localization of lymphoid cells.* Ser Haematol 8:482, 1974.

SUPPRESSOR CELLS:

WALDMANN TA, BLAESE RM, BRODER S, ET AL: *Disorders of suppressor immunoregulatory cells in the pathogenesis of immunodeficiency and autoimmunity.* Ann Intern Med 88:226, 1978.

IMMUNOGLOBULINS:

NATVIG JB, AND KUNKEL HG: *Human immunoglobulins: Classes, subclasses genetic variants and idiotypes.* Adv Immunol 16:1, 1973.

SOLOMON A, AND MCLAUGHLIN CL: *Immunoglobulin structure determined from products of plasma cell neoplasms.* Semin Hematol 10:3, 1973.

SPIEGELBERG HL: *Biological activities of immunoglobulins of different classes and subclasses.* Adv Immunol 19:259, 1974.

WALDMAN RH, AND GANGULY R: *Role of immune mechanisms on secretory surfaces in prevention of infection.* In Allen (ed): *Infection and the Compromised Host.* Williams & Wilkins, Baltimore, 1976, p 29.

LYMPHOCYTIC NEOPLASMS:

BERARD CW, GREENE MH, JAFFE ES, ET AL: *A multidisciplinary approach to non-Hogkin's lymphomas.* Ann Intern Med 94:218, 1981.

LUTZNER M, EDELSON R, SCHEIN P, ET AL: *Cutaneous T-cell lymphomas: The Sezary syndrome, mycosis fungoides, and related disorders.* Ann Intern Med 83:534, 1975.

The non-Hodgkin's lymphoma pathologic classification project. National Cancer Institute-sponsored study of classification of non-Hodgkin's lymphoma. Cancer 49:2112, 1982.

IMMUNOGENETICS:

MANN DL, AND MURRAY C: *HLA alloantigens: Disease association and biological significance.* Semin Hematol 16:293, 1979.

MILLER WV: *The human histocompatibility complex: A review for the hematologist.* Prog Hematol 10:173, 1977.

INDEX

A "t" indicates a table.
An *italic* number indicates a figure.

Disease(s)
  acute lymphoblastic leukemia, 89
  associated with abnormal T-cell
    subsets, 72, t
  autoimmune, 71–72
  B-cell malignancy, 89, *90*
  chronic granulomatous, 45
  chronic lymphocytic leukemia, 89
  common variable gammaglobulinemia,
    88
  complement deficiency, 45–46
  DiGeorge's, 64, 86–87
  Gaucher's, 54
  graft-versus-host, 68
  histiocytosis X, 53
  Hodgkin's, 24, 95–96
  immune deficiency, 86–97
  kinetic changes in, 34–38
  leukemia, 15–18
  lymphoid lymphoma, 93
  macroglobulinemia, 92–93
  monocyte-macrophage system and,
    53–54
  multiple myeloma, 91
  selective absence of IgA, 88
  severe combined immunodeficiency,
    86–87
  X-linked agammaglobulinemia, 87
DNA, stem cells and, 8–9
Drug(s)
  antitumor, 27–28
  cytotoxic, 38

ENDOCYTOSIS, killing cascade and, 41
Enzymes
  lymphocytes and, 78–80
  immune deficiency syndromes and,
    79–80
Eosinopenia
  detection of, 54–55
  inflammatory processes and, 55
Eosinophilia, 54
Eosinophil(s)
  allergic reactions and, 56–57, t
  compared with neutrophils, 54, 56
  components of, 56
  described, 4, 54
  effectiveness of, 56
  function of, 55
  idiopathic forms of, 57
  schistosomiasis and, 55–56

GAMMAGLOBULIN, 83. *See also*
    Immunoglobulin.
Gout, neutrophils and, 46, 48

HAPLOTYPE, 97. *See also*
    Immunogenetics.
Hematopoiesis
  extramedullary, 13–15
  myeloid, 13
Hemodialysis, neutrophils and, 48
Histiocyte(s), as synonym for
    macrophage, 53
Histocytic medullary reticulosis, 53
Histiocytosis X, 53
Hodgkin's disease
  clinical features of, 24, 95–96
  course of, 24
  monocyte-macrophage system and,
    53
  Reed-Sternberg cells and, 95
  treatment of, 24
HSC compartment(s), 9. *See also* Stem
    cell system.

IMMUNE defense system, function of,
    62–63
Immune deficiency disease(s)
  primary, 86–88
    common variable
      hypogammaglobulinemia, 88
    DiGeorge's syndrome, 86–87
    selective absence of IgA, 88
    severe combined, 86
    X-linked agammaglobulinemia, 87
  secondary, 88–95
    acute lymphoblastic leukemia, 89
    B-cell malignancy and, 89
    chronic lymphocytic leukemia, 89–
      90
    lymphoid lymphomas, 93, *94,* 95
    macroglobulinemia, 92–93
    monoclonal gamopathies, benign,
      93
    multiple myeloma, 91–92
    T-cell lymphoma, 95
Immune reactivity, *71*
Immunocyte system, mechanisms of,
    1–2
Immunogenetics
  chromosome #6 and, *96*
  haplotype and, 97

Migration
  chemotaxins and, 39, *40*, 41
  defects of, 45–46
  neutrophils and, *14*, 38–39
  tests for integrity of, 39
Mitogens, lymphocytes and, 77
Mitosis
  hepatocytes and, 9
  neutrophils and, 32
  neutrophil precursors and, 4
  process of, described, 7, *8*
  progenitor cells and, 11
Monoclonal antibodies
  production of, 70–71
  use in tracing cell maturation, 72, *73*
Monocyte(s), described, 5, 49
Monocyte-macrophage system
  disease and, 53–54
  function of, 50–53
    cellular activation, 51
    cleaning, 52–53
    immunologic, 51
    microbiocidal, 51–52
  terminology describing, 49
Multiple myeloma
  major features of, 91
  protein abnormalities in, 91, t, 92
  renal failure and, 92
Myeloblasts, 3
Myelocytes, 3
Myeloid
  defined, 9
  end-stage cells and, 12
  HSC system and, 9–10, *12*
Myeloid leukemia
  acute, 20–23
    cell production in, 22
    malignancy of, 20–21
    mortality, 23
    physical findings in, 2
    treatment of, 22–23
  chronic, 19–20
    clinical features of, 19–20
    mechanism of neutrophil production
      in, 22
    pathogenesis of, 20
    Philadelphia chromosome and, 19–
      20

NEOPLASM(S). *See also* Stem cell
  disease.

clonal, 15–25
  classified, 15, 17, t
  G6PD analysis and, 15, *16*
  leukemia and, 15–16
  X-chromosomes and, 15
  macrophages and, 52
Neutropenia
  cytotoxic drugs and, 38
  fever and, 38
  neutrophil dysfunction and, 38
  types of, 37, t
Neutrophil(s)
  adverse effects of, 46, 48
  band, described, 3
  chemotaxins and, 39, *40,* 41
  defects of, 45–46
    alternate pathway to avoid, *46*
    factors influencing concentration of,
      34
  function of, 29–30, 38
    migration cascade and, 38–39
  killing capacity of, 45
  kinetics of, 30, *31, 32*
    infection and, 34, *35*
    interpretation of changes in, 36
  locomotion of, 41
  margination of, 30, 38
  maturation of, 3, 33
  morphologic abnormalities of, 48–49
  morphology of, *33*
  neutropenia and, 38
  production and storage of, 32–34
    mitotic pool and, 32
    postmitotic pool and, 32
  studies of, 30, 31
NK cells, function of, 76
Null cells, described, 75–76

PAROXYSMAL nocturnal hemoglobinuria,
  24
Pelger-Huet anomaly, described, 49
Phagocyte system
  bone marrow and, 30–*32*
  function of, 29
  neutrophils and, 29–34
Phagocytosis, biochemical process of, 2,
  42, *43, 44*
Philadelphia chromosome, 19–20
Plasma cells, described, 5
PMN. *See* Neutrophils.
Polycemia vera